Stop Surviving,
Start Thriving

Find Your Perfect Balance in a Not-So-Perfect World

KIM ROBINSON NETO

Stop Surviving, Start Thriving:
Find Your Perfect Balance in a Not-So-Perfect World

Copyright © 2015 by Kim Robinson Neto

Disclaimer
The content of this book is for general instruction only. Each person's physical, emotional, and spiritual condition is unique. The instruction in this book is not intended to replace or interrupt the reader's relationship with a physician or other professional. Always consult a qualified doctor or medical practitioners for matters pertaining to your specific health and diet.

To contact the publisher, visit:
www.simplewellnesswithkim.com
SIMPLE WELLNESS
Castro Valley, CA

ISBN-13: 978-0692415344
ISBN-10: 978-0692415343

Library of Congress Control Number: 2015905394
First Edition

Printed in the United States of America

Praise for *Stop Surviving, Start Thriving*

"*Stop Surviving, Start Thriving* is a must-read book for busy women who are stressed out and frazzled with too much on their plates. This book is packed with practical tips on how to reduce stress, practice better self-care, and enjoy life to the fullest! Kim Robinson Neto shares her simple yet powerful strategies in such an engaging manner; reading this book is like having a conversation with a very wise and health-conscious friend."

> ~ Tiffany deSilva, MSW, CPC, CHC, author of *Fantastically Free* and *BrightFire Living*

"Kim's words brilliantly echo the experiences of many women. *Stop Surviving, Start Thriving* is that voice of reason that busy women seek in order to give themselves permission to make healthy changes. Read it as a gift to yourself, your family, your friends!"

> ~ Melanie Banayat, author of *Stretch Your Brave Hack Your Story; Break Through Chronic Disease with Storytelling*

"The title says it all! In *Stop Surviving, Start Thriving* Kim Robinson Neto has written a wonderful plan of action that teaches readers how to navigate the potentially frustrating and overwhelming process of being a mom, raising a family in the sandwich generation, while taking care of elderly parents. Kim tells the story of going from the depths of despair by living a life on overwhelm into revealing the secrets behind living a mindful, more balanced, healthy life."

> ~ Elaine Lombardi, CHHC, AADP, author of *Hurricane Lucy: A Caregiver's Guide Navigating the Storm of Caring for Your Aging Parent*

To my amazing son, Evan.
I love you to the moon and back.

In memory of my parents, Jack and Teresita.
I miss them every single day.

♥

And to all the women who have given up their lives to care
for others, may this book inspire and nourish you.

Table of Contents

PART THREE
Love Yourself

PART FOUR
Tools for Thriving

Acknowledgements

There are so many people who have been a part of my healing that I can't possibly name everyone. Their presence contributed to my spiritual growth, my happiness, mental well-being and physical health. I have many people to thank for just being in my life. I dedicate this book to my parents, Jack and Teresita, who gave me the foundation for all that I am today. Although they have passed on, their presence is in my heart always. *A special thank you to:* Clarence McCurdy and Valentine Armstrong for giving me life, giving me love, and believing in me. Paul for working hard so I can follow my dreams, Maria and Eliseu Neto for always coming to my rescue, Tita Rosie for being my favorite aunt, my sister Rachel for being my voice of reason, my beautiful niece Delena Armstrong for being my first client. Also, I thank Susan Green my accountability partner and healthy friend, my longtime BFF's; Kelly, Cynthia, Kathy, Rosa (Lupita), Pam, and Margie for keeping me sane and grounded, and my wonderful mom friends; Kim O., Melissa, Amy, Rieko, Rachel, Bonnie, Sylvia, Alpana, Nadia, Rachael, and Kathryn for being such supportive women. Thanks also to Cherlynn Thomas for her useful ideas, Sylvia Martinez-Banks and Kellee Louderback-Gibson for their valuable feedback, my graphic designer Kay at Bookdesign for my beautiful cover and my editor Jennifer Barrows for catching my mistakes. And to Joshua Rosenthal, Lindsey Smith and all my peers at the Institute for Integrative Nutrition for pushing me to keep writing and get this book published!

Finally, a very special thank you to my son Evan, for inspiring me to take care of myself and my health. (Thank you for putting up with mommy always being on the computer)

Introduction

Over the years, I've watched many of my friends struggle with their weight and health as they grew older and raised families. Their stories aren't unusual. Because in today's world, women are doing more than ever. Whether you are a full-time stay-at-home mom, part-time working mom, full-time career woman, or empty nester, you are either in the throes of keeping everything together or have put in a great amount of work raising your family and you are left dealing with poor health. However you got to this point, starting this moment, you are taking the first step toward improving your health and your life. If you follow my suggestions in this book and make simple changes over time, you will be amazed at how incredible you will feel in just a short time.

You may be wondering what makes me an expert on surviving and thriving in this world. I decided to write this book as the result of my two year journey back to health; a healing journey that I took after a very stressful and challenging time in my life. At my lowest point, I felt so disconnected from my body that it was almost as if I really wasn't alive. Every day felt as though I was just surviving. I was making it through one more day, without joy or happiness, but rather with pain and suffering. Moving from surviving to thriving has left me feeling more energetic and alive than I did in my 30s. Now in midlife, I have made it past the first half of my life; through the highs and lows, the ups and downs, the joy and sorrow, all life's experiences that come from living fifty years on this earth. With gratitude, I survived. Perhaps my story is similar to yours, or maybe not. But what we both have in common is that I am a *real* woman and have daily challenges just like you. I'm not perfect and it's taken me years to finally reach a healthy balance in my life. And now I want to share what I have learned with you.

I wrote this book as a simple guide you can read quickly and use as a reference. Being a busy woman, I understand you don't have time to read through pages and pages of information. So this book cuts straight to the core. No added fluff, just practical and useful advice. I hope to show you how simple it can be to return to health despite having a crazy life. My intention is to introduce you to changes you can make every day that will add up to big results in the quality of your life. Wouldn't you like to live a long and healthy life? I sure do! I'm a believer that what you do today will make an impact on your life tomorrow. I'm an advocate for everything in moderation. I won't tell you that you can never enjoy your favorite foods again, or that you need to spend hours breaking a sweat in the gym. I want to show you how to enjoy life and still have control over your food and lifestyle choices. I'm here to tell you that being born a woman does not mean you are destined to gain weight as you age, feel exhausted all the time, or suffer with joint pain and osteoporosis. I want you to know that you do have the power to a live a healthy and fulfilling life. And it's my hope that this book will inspire you to go for it!

I tell my clients to imagine what their life could be like if they woke up each morning with energy and excitement for the day. How about *you*? What would you do differently if you didn't suffer from exhaustion, headaches, anxiety or poor digestion? What have you been dreaming to accomplish? How would you feel if you *really* loved the person you saw in the mirror each day? You would feel amazing, that's for sure. Let me say congratulations to beautiful YOU. By reading this book, you are making a positive step to improve your life. My wish is that after reading through the chapters and making simple changes in your life, you will feel healthier and happier than you ever have, with a new excitement for food and a new passion for living. That you will stop running in survival mode and start to *thrive*.

PART ONE
The Balancing Act

"My mission in life is not merely to survive, but to thrive;
and to do so with some passion, some compassion, some humor,
and some style."

— *Maya Angelou*

Chapter 1
My Story

Many years ago, when my son was born, I was wrapped in a blanket of warm and fuzzy feelings mixed with fear and anxiety. I was a new mom, and here was this little soul who depended on me for safety, security and unconditional love. It was a huge departure from my former life as a free spirited woman with a successful career, who could come and go as she pleases. I always had time to go out with friends, exercise at any hour, and find plenty of opportunities to spend time by myself. If anything happened to me, there was no little person who would be left motherless. No guilty feelings if I wanted to stay out late, drink wine and drive fast. Yet, becoming a mother changed all of that in an instant. I had no option to try it out, ease into motherhood, or slowly wean myself from having alone time. It was a change that I never gave much thought about, until it happened.

Of course, there is nothing more fulfilling than looking into the eyes of your precious baby and feeling overwhelming love. But in that very moment, my life was no longer about me. It was as if, through some natural maternal instinct, my needs didn't matter anymore. I was ready to do whatever was necessary to make this tiny human being thrive. If it meant that I didn't sleep for 48 hours, so be it. It didn't matter if I ate healthy food, slept a full eight hours or saw another person. In those first months of motherhood, all that mattered in this world was my baby.

If only I knew. Knew that the moment he was born, my life would change then, and in all the years to come. Nothing could have prepared me for the journey of motherhood and all the responsibility that came with raising a family. It wasn't too long after my son was born that I realized just how much of my free time disappeared. Like every new mother, we start to pay attention and realize, hey, my needs have dropped to the bottom of the list. Many sleepless nights became a part of my everyday life, and meals were whatever food I could find within my reach. Which usually meant I was eating sodium filled takeout food or anything edible out of a can.

Those early years, I also started to experience emotions than I never knew existed. I loved having this bundle of joy to love and hold, (and I actually surprised myself with what a great job I was doing) but what I didn't expect was that I would end up feeling so tired and wired at the same time. Who knew that raising a child, running a household and keeping it all together would be the hardest job I ever had. Wasn't motherhood supposed to be all about bear hugs and kisses?

This new role of "superwoman" just seemed to land in my lap. I really didn't have a vote in my own election. I remember secretly envying other moms when they talked about their husbands watching the baby so they could go and do something nice for themselves. I just didn't have that option. My husband worked long hours and wasn't interested in watching the baby on the weekends. In fact, he would frequently sleep until lunchtime and have no problem checking out mentally on his days off. But there were no days off for me. I had to suck it up, not complain and be that "superwoman" to keep everything moving like clockwork. No time to rest, no time to relax, and barely time to go to the bathroom!

It was never in my life plan to stay home with a child. But the first day I went back to my office job, after an extended maternity leave, it became clear I would give up my career to stay at home and be with my baby. It's a decision I will never, ever regret. I looked at my role as a stay-at-home mom (SAHM) as my new full-time job. A very special job too, with the kind of satisfaction you would never get from working at a company. And truthfully, I didn't mind living in sweatpants and tee shirts all day. (THE most comfortable clothing, right moms?) I also didn't need to spend an hour in the bathroom styling my hair or putting on makeup. On most days it was easiest to just throw my long locks into a pony tail and go. Yes, I had become the classic stay at home mom, complete with the very safe, very boring, Volvo station wagon.

My life as a mom was plugging along and it was actually getting fun watching my toddler hit his milestones. The fun, was in large part due to the wonderful support of my local Mom's group. Without the regular social time for moms, as well as for the kids, I could see how easily it would have been to become isolated or worse, fall into a depression. But little did I know an even bigger challenge was just down the road that would turn my life upside down. A time when my life would really get complicated. A time I would start to just survive, and no longer thrive.

It happened around the time my son hit his terrible threes. My mother's health started declining and the time had come when my parent's seriously needed my help. Always being the responsible daughter, I naturally began to take over their care. And there I was, driving back and forth 30 miles to my parent's house in the city while dragging along my screaming toddler. I'm not sure why it never occurred to me that this would happen. I'd heard about the so called "sandwich generation" where you are old enough to have senior parents yet young enough to have dependent children of your own. It had never entered my mind that I would be stuck in this situation. Almost overnight, it became my responsibility to handle the care of my parents while raising my own child. It was during this period of my life that I felt helpless for the first time. I had always thought of myself as a strong and capable woman, yet with so many obligations pulling me in every direction, my life started spiraling out of control. I found myself worrying about everyone's health except mine. Then my life reached a point where feeling out of balance was all I knew. And for the first time, I started to feel really sick.

This was a strange place for me.

You see, I was lucky to have been adopted and raised by parents who valued health and eating real food. They never bought into the 1970s craze of Swanson's TV dinners, Oscar Meyer bologna or Frosted Flakes cereal. Our family was not a typical family growing up during the birth of plastic packaging and highly processed foods; a time when Pepsi and Coke replaced milk, and everyone loved eating Hamburger Helper. Not us. We sat around the table serving real, fresh, home cooked food. My grandmother would spend all day in the kitchen preparing wholesome meals that I would later come to appreciate. I'm more thankful now, for learning the foundation of what a healthy meal should look like. Not out of a box, a can, or a package, but grown in the ground, picked from a tree, or found on a real farm.

Being raised on a relatively healthy diet and having a father who was obsessed with exercise was a part of my daily existence. I lived without aches and pains. I didn't know what it felt like to be tired for no reason. I had no clue what it felt like to function on less than abundant energy. Watching my body break down and my energy disappear while under so much stress, was a totally foreign feeling for me. It was at this point that I started to realize that something was very wrong. The years of constant worry over my parents, plus raising a young child and never being able to get a good night's sleep or take a moment to breathe, was slowly stealing my health and wellness. I knew in my heart that something had to change, but I didn't feel in control. My body was becoming sick, my mind fuzzy and I felt completely powerless. If I couldn't change my life circumstance, how could I climb out of this terrible hole?

I remember it started with fatigue in the afternoon. A feeling of being so tired that I could only lie on the sofa and stare at the blank TV. Getting up to make dinner felt like an impossibly daunting task, and over time, these lethargic episodes would happen more and more frequently. I started to turn to caffeine, only to learn quickly it wasn't the answer. The running back and forth to hospitals, nursing homes, doctor's offices, playdates and volunteering at my son's school, became an exhausting routine for me. I remember driving to the hospital one day, looking out at the other people going about their day, and thinking, will I ever feel like a normal person again? I couldn't even remember what it felt like to be worry free or to wake up without my mind racing with anxious thoughts. Would I ever be able to just have a normal day, where all I needed to worry about was what to make for dinner and not if something terrible would happen? I thought to myself, "is this the beginning of the end?" Here I was in my 40s and already feeling like life was almost over!

I tried to convince myself that everything happening was just a part of growing old. After all, I had plenty of friends my age that were complaining of similar types of health worries. Didn't all 40-year-olds have chronic headaches, feel exhausted, be anxious and wake up with aches and pains? Maybe you've heard the phrase, "misery loves company" well, we were all feeling sick and tired, and secretly, I was happy to know it wasn't just me.

Besides the exhaustion, I was also suffering from frequent migraines and debilitating panic attacks. My panic attacks were happening so frequently I became a prisoner in my own home. Whenever my husband left for work, the panic would set in, and I often felt as if I wouldn't survive until he came back. One day, my worst nightmare happened. My father had a serious fall that sent him the ER. It wasn't his first time to the emergency room by any means, but it would be the last time he left his house. The next four months were filled with worry, anxiety and intense emotions that would drain every ounce of energy from my body. Each day that I sat with my father in the hospital knowing his days in this life were nearing an end, I was also overcome with guilt, knowing my son was somewhere missing his mommy. During those last months leading up to my father's death, my mental stability and physical health nearly reached their breaking point. But nothing could prepare me for what happened only two months later, when my mother took a turn for the worse and would also pass away, leaving my sister and me as orphans. Just like that.

In the year after my parents' passing, my stress level continued to rage on. Having to handle the estate, distributing the family assets, selling the home, and taking care of every detail, was an emotionally and physically challenging time. Once the final papers were signed and my parent's belongings were all settled, I finally started to emerge as a new person. It's ironic how death seems to bring life. The deep sadness that comes with losing someone close to you can also bring forth an opportunity for growth. The experience I endured while caring for my parents, the doctor visits, medical treatments and watching them become frail, had actually inspired me to improve my own life. I knew it was time to heal my body and mind, and focus on being the best role model to my son. The kitchen became the heart of my house. If I could nourish my body with nutritious food, maybe I could heal from the effects of all my stress. I couldn't control life or the need to keep putting out fires, but the choice of what to put into my body was mine. All mine. And it was the one thing I *could* control. So I started to fill my shopping basket with fresh produce and real (unprocessed) food—despite the resistance from my husband and son. It became my personal mission to eat healthier, live better and nourish my body, if they liked it or not.

The healthy food was a good start, but something else was still missing in my life. The nourishment helped to balance the effects of my stress, but it wasn't enough. I was feeding my body, but I also needed to nourish my soul. With my parents gone, the door had been opened to work on outside relationships again. No longer busy with running from here to there, I could finally slow down and take an inventory of the people in my life. Spending time with lost friends and new friends restored my spirit, as did reconnecting with my biological parents. I had found them years before, but was never able to devote energy to growing our relationship. I felt blessed to have been given a second chance to know unconditional love from the two individuals who gave me life. Never a replacement for the parents who raised me, but a very special bond with two very special people.

You've probably heard the expression, "It's never too late." What a wonderful statement it is. Because, I truly believe it is never too late to do anything that will improve your life. Shortly after the dust had settled, I received an email in my inbox. It was a message from a school I had never heard of, but yet was the largest nutrition school in the country. The timing seemed perfect. How did this holistic healing institution know it was exactly what I needed? When that email reached my inbox, I was about to hit midlife. Old enough to feel like I should be planning my retirement and not starting a new career. But somehow, I was captivated. I always had a passion for health and wellness, so the possibility piqued my interest. I put any doubts aside and followed my heart. The very next day I called the school for an interview, was accepted and enrolled. Everything in my body and soul had been screaming "go for it!" so I did.

Over the next year, I studied holistic health and nutrition and learned to find my own perfect balance. My life was growing in ways I never expected. I began to exercise more and started practicing yoga. I reflected on my life and began healing inside. I was happier, hopeful and my spirit was lifted. I had found a community of like-minded individuals on a similar journey. I no longer felt drawn to plop on the sofa and space out, instead my feet would march outside and do something healthy and fun. I look back and realize that there were two major changes that saved my life. Learning to nourish my body with the right foods and finding peace and calm through yoga. These two simple, yet very powerful changes gave my mind and body a new beginning.

It isn't a coincidence they say there is a mind-body connection. You need a healthy mind to have a healthy body.

Graduating from the Institute for Integrative Nutrition and becoming a health coach gave me overwhelming satisfaction. I am grateful to have found my passion in life. Being able to help other women live a longer and happier life is priceless. I have had the pleasure of working with many women in their midlife, who have actually taught me some valuable life lessons. One client, a 78 year old woman, decided it was her time to take back her health. I am always amazed. Proof that you can never be too old to change your life. She was so interested in health that she learned more about natural supplements and healing foods than most of the younger women I know. And I know some really healthy women!

Whatever your story may be, either single, married, divorced, kids, or no kids, you have the ability to take control of your health right now and make the decision to live your best life possible. No matter what age you are, know that you are on the road to a healthier and happier life. One of my favorite quotes is by Lao Tzu, and says "A journey of a thousand miles begins with a single step." It's such a profound, yet simple statement. It encourages me to embrace change and keep moving forward.

If you look at your life with only one beginning and one end, it probably feels like it's all over. The truth is we have many beginnings and many endings. That's the nature of life. When you feel discouraged and overwhelmed in your current day-to-day life, remember the words of Lao Tzu. Because each new day is a chance to begin a new journey. I wouldn't want it any other way.

"Rock bottom became a solid foundation for which I rebuilt my life"
- Unknown

Chapter 2
Too Much on Your Plate

If you are reading this book, you are probably the one who does everything in your family. You are like a silent saint who is holding everything together. You have somehow found yourself in a role of the primary caretaker, and now you are stuck. And if you were to stop doing everything you do for just one day, your home would probably look like a tornado ran through it! Don't feel bad, you are in the same sinking ship as the majority of women in this country. It isn't unusual to have female friends in your life who take care of the kids, husband, parents, dogs, cats, birds, and all the household chores. And sometimes that's in addition to having a full-time career.

I'm sure you can remember your own mother or grandmother being the matriarch of their homes. As women, it's almost as though we are hardwired to give so much of ourselves. We give and give and give. We do everything for our children. We stress over keeping the house clean. We want to please our parents. We cater to our husbands. We try to be great friends. We worry about what to make for breakfast, lunch and dinner. And we get up every morning even though we are exhausted to do it all over again. If you could climb into a time machine and go back a thousand years, you would see women taking care of the children, helping the elders, preparing food, tending to the home and being the rock of the family structure. But you don't really need a time machine, because today you can walk into any history museum and there you will see images of women tending to the babies, preparing food, fetching water or weaving baskets and making clay cooking pots. From the beginning of time, women have been the backbone of human existence. We have been the caretakers during each generation of life.

I often wonder why women give so much of themselves. We do this even if we didn't learn it from our mothers and grandmothers. It's no wonder that science has shown that women use more areas of the grey matter in the brain and are more sensitive to emotions and negativity than men. Perhaps this is why we tend to be more caring, compassionate and nurturing. And may also explain why women are more prone to anxiety and depression. Unfortunately, this hard wired tendency to take care of everyone and everything leaves us feeling burned out and depressed. I personally, have watched many women struggle with just staying afloat every day. We seem to take on more than we should, yet keep on going no matter what the consequences. We would rather wear ourselves out, sacrifice our time, and get sick rather than feel like we are imposing on others for help.

I know a woman who spends all of her time taking care of her husband and two teenaged kids. She barely has a social life outside her home and is the classic housewife in every sense. She does all the cooking, cleaning, grocery shopping, laundry, and takes care of all the family needs. When her kids were young, she helped with their homework, made medical appointments and volunteered at their schools. Is this woman starting to sound familiar? If it isn't you, I'm sure you can think of at least one woman in your life who fits this description.

The first step toward a more balanced life is to acknowledge that you have too much on your plate. Do you really need to do everything? You may feel as if you have to, that no one else is capable of doing what you do, but you need to learn to let go and start making room for the things in your life that nourish you. I encourage you to make a list of everything you do. Look at it carefully. What can you cross off? What can you hand over to your husband or partner? Can you hire someone else to do it?

If you are an all or nothing kind of gal, this is especially important for you. Trying to be a perfectionist in all areas of your life is only going to make life harder. Ask yourself what would happen if you didn't put all of your heart and soul into one task. It's okay to do just enough to get by. It really is. It took me some time and practice to be able to lower my standards, so that I didn't feel like whatever I was doing had to be perfect. If your plate is overflowing and everything on that plate has to be done perfectly, how is that productive? What ends up happening is that nothing gets done and you are still busy. That's certainly not the way to be productive!

It can be eye opening to learn just how much we actually do each day. Until I sat down and wrote out a list of all the tasks that I took care of in a typical day, did I see how much I do in comparison to my husband. It also helped me to see all the tasks I do which are not very important. I encourage you to give it a try. This exercise may be eye opening for you too. Your goal is to see how much you do and find ways to simplify your life. Cross things off your list that can be done less often, or even at all. Maybe something you do can be handled by someone else? This is an excellent exercise to try with your spouse or partner. Have them make a list too and work on sharing responsibilities. You may also realize just how much inequity is happening in your family, as I did.

Sometimes we end up with husbands who are unwilling or incapable to share the burden of raising kids and running a household. If you happen to find yourself in this situation, it's important to look closely at your life. Too many women find themselves stuck in the traditional (and sexist) role of taking care of everything and everyone. Until we acknowledge that we can't continue to do it all, we will be forever living with frustration and anger. If this is you, it's time to take a serious look at your life and make a move to get unstuck.

Clear Your Plate

1. Take a sheet of paper and list the things you do in an average day. Be sure to list everything, making the bed, walking the dog, driving kids to school, working on a project, preparing dinner and even changing the cat litter. Write everything down that you do!

2. On a separate sheet of paper, make two columns: MUST and MAYBE.

3. From your list of responsibilities, write each item into one of the columns. When you have finished moving everything over, look at your list.

4. Tasks under the MUST column should be things that absolutely have to be done, like take the kids to school or make dinner. Everything else that is not crucial can be MAYBE. Those are the things that won't cause life to come crashing down if they don't get done.

5. Look at your new list. Is there anything else you can move to the MAYBE side?

6. Now, what can you hand over to your spouse or kids? It's time to divide the chores that are on the MUST list.

7. Use this list as a tool to map out your week. Perhaps some of the items on your daily list can be done on a weekly basis.

The Superwoman Syndrome

If you are old enough to remember the 1970s and 80s, it was the peak of the women's movement. To be an independent woman was every young girl's dream. I still remember a television commercial for a perfume called Enjoli. This iconic clip featured a catchy jingle that went, "cause I'm a woman, I can bring home the bacon, fry it up in a pan, and never let you forget you're a man." Does it ring a bell? It was quite popular, and I'm sure I wasn't the only person walking around in the 80's singing this catchy tune. Of course, advertisements are intentionally created around a trend, so this commercial probably helped sprout a new generation of women. As a young woman in my 20's, I watched some of my own friends try to have this "ideal" life, working at a job, raising kids, being the sexy wife, keeping a tidy house and trying to look fabulous. But, as many women learned, it's impossible to be this 24 hour woman. Because that's exactly how many hours you would need to get everything done!

Honestly, if this sounds familiar, you can't keep running full speed ahead, pleasing everyone and doing everything. Sure, you can keep running around and being superwoman for several years, but unless you plan to start seeing your doctor frequently, you need to slow down. Rushing around and doing everything will eventually make you sick. And I mean really sick. As in chronic illness or worse. You are setting yourself up for a difficult last half of your life. I know you don't want that! I'm not trying to scare you, rather make a point that there are consequences with trying to be a superwoman. Trust me, that person just doesn't exist. You are a woman with needs. Which means you don't have to please everyone. Taking care of yourself is the best thing you can do to come closer to feeling like a superwoman.

If what I'm saying has your attention, then please listen carefully. **It's time to stop taking care of everything and everyone.** It took me a long time to let this sink into my own life. Yes, I realize that may mean the dishes don't always get washed, or the laundry will pile up, or the crumbs on the floor will make a feast for the ants. But really, in the grander scheme of life, everyone will survive. I'm not suggesting that you stop feeding the kids (although the older ones can handle their own breakfast and make lunches) but you have to draw the line somewhere. What I am suggesting you do is delegate or let things go. As much as we feel like we are the only one in the family capable of doing everything right, we aren't. I know this. Why? Because your family members have hands, feet and a brain, right? They are capable of pitching in and helping out. If you want to feel like Superwoman, then it's time to ask your husband, partner and kids to do their share.

Okay, so everyone probably won't jump to their feet and wait for your orders. Unless you are lucky enough to have an amazing husband and eager kids. But if you're like most of us, it might take many conversations and much patience. It took me months and months of feeling resentment, anger, and frustration before some of the simplest tasks got done without my constant nagging. And to be honest, even after many years, I still have to remind my husband of his weekly task to take out the garbage. But even that one task is one less thing I have to do. Every family is different, including yours, so delegate the chores you can't (or don't want to) handle and go from there. The more willing your family members are to help out, the happier and healthier you will be in the long run.

If you wait for things to change on their own, you may be waiting a very long time. Unless you have a mind reader in the family, no one will know how you are feeling. I tried the wait and see game for years and it only made me more frustrated, more tired and depressed. Trying to be the martyr will only make your life unhappy, because ultimately you are the one who is left drained and exhausted. So don't let yourself fall into this trap. As women, we tend to keep going, taking care of everyone, and feeling frustrated. We don't complain, and when we do, we forgive quickly and forget. And then we keep doing everything and nothing changes. Remember, it's your life, and unless you speak up and choose to change a situation, the same routine will keep going on forever.

After reaching my breaking point (many times) and making ultimatums, things would change for a while. Having a husband who isn't very domestic around the house and not wired the same as me, created a greater challenge than most. If only men would understand that women want a partner who demonstrate their love by pitching in around the house, rather than giving a bouquet of roses or an expensive necklace and then sitting on the couch with their feet up. But I know why men choose to give gifts over doing the dishes, it's so much easier! They only need to walk into a store and buy a gift, rather than helping with housework for a month. Or, at least until their wives start complaining again. Well, we women know differently, right! The fastest way to a woman's heart is for a man to do his share of work around the house. Give her a day off from the kids and send her to the spa! That would make any woman feel loved. (I'm sure many of you are nodding your heads right now!) Perhaps it's time to stop hinting and start talking. It's time to get rid of any buried resentment.

Here is my challenge to you. I want you to start delegating some tasks this week. If you need to make this fun, why not create a chore wheel. Play it like a game and let everyone take a spin. Maybe even have a space for "free time" so your kids won't be discouraged. Remember, dividing up the housework will make your life easier. You can start with simple tasks for the younger ones and more complicated chores for the adults. Over time, you can simply add tasks as the kids grow older. This is also a great opportunity for everyone to see just how much you do every day!

If a chore wheel isn't your thing, you can always just assign tasks and rotate every week. That's what my family did when I was growing up. I still remember we all hated to vacuum and wash dishes. Rotating chores made it feel more equitable between us three kids. If you have a small family or are a single mom, another strategy is to just give up some of the daily chores. This is what worked for me. Since my husband couldn't take on much and my son was still young, I looked at everything I did every day and began crossing chores off my list. I asked myself if I really needed to clean the bathrooms more than once a week? Was it going to hurt anyone if the dishes sat in the sink overnight? Could we survive a few days or a week without doing laundry? Sure, I would love to have the perfect home, but for every hour I spent cleaning, meant time away from doing something more meaningful and nourishing for *me*.

Think about your own life. What can you cross off your list that will give you more time during the day, or the week, to do something nurturing like getting a massage or having tea with a friend. I completely understand if you're a super organized person. Yes, it will be hard to let things go. If you can afford it, hire a cleaning person. After taking a cue from another busy mom, I hired a woman to clean my house and boy did it help. I had a beautiful clean home for about two days. It was a glorious, chore free two days! And when you are a busy, stressed-out woman, even two days of rest feels like a vacation. If money is tight in your family, or you just don't feel comfortable with a stranger in your house, then it's time to let some of the chores go. When I realized our budget could no longer afford a regular cleaning person, I started letting my house look a little messy. Admittedly, it left me feeling frustrated at first. But the free time I enjoyed was priceless. Instead of scrubbing down all three of our bathrooms, I was able to spend quality time with my son, or go for a peaceful hike with the dog. I learned how to straighten up, rather than deep clean, and accepted that my house doesn't have to look perfect all the time. It was difficult at first, but I encourage you to try it. Maybe just a little. If a neat freak like me can change, so can you! When you can let go of perfection, you will be a much happier person.

Women are naturally multi-taskers, pleasers, and doers. We are not lazy. We are good at getting things done quick and efficiently. But this is also why we are more prone to anxiety and depression. We take on more than we should and don't complain. If we can learn to let go of tasks and ask for help, we start to honor our time and our health. Ultimately, the goal is to find more time to do the things we really enjoy. Something that is nourishing and meaningful to our life. It could be taking a walk in nature, playing with a child, going shopping, visiting a museum, or having tea with a friend. If you are someone who happens to find washing the dishes therapeutic, then by all means keep doing it! Just don't feel guilty asking for help with the tedious chores you don't like, such as taking out the garbage, like me. Resist the urge to do something yourself just so it's perfect. You don't need to make it right. If your husband loads the dishwasher all wrong, it's okay. The dishes will still get clean. If he vacuums around the furniture or cleans the toilet with bath tissue, relax, it isn't the end of the world. Remember, you don't have to act like a superhero to be Superwoman. Anyway, superheroes don't do housework!

Physical Symptoms of Superwoman Syndrome (aka Stress)

- Headaches, especially migraines
- Fatigued, feeling tired all the time
- Anxious, irritable, moody
- Panic attacks
- Insomnia and trouble staying asleep
- Weight gain or weight loss
- Digestive issues; constipation, diarrhea, IBS
- Hormonal imbalance; irregular menstrual cycles
- Increased heart rate (resting over 80 BPM)
- Chest pain or angina
- Palpitations, irregular heart beats
- GERD or chronic indigestion
- Elevated blood pressure
- Elevated blood sugar
- Ringing in the ears
- Shallow breathing
- Dizziness
- Foggy brain, trouble concentrating, forgetful

Chapter 3
Motherhood

There comes a point in time when every woman wonders if she will become a mother. Some women are born with this burning desire and feel as if their lives would never be complete without a house full of happy kids running around. Some women imagine being a mother someday, but decide to build their career first. Some women start their families and put careers on hold. And, some women just accept that motherhood is not for them. No matter what kind of woman you are, you are a natural caregiver. We are born that way.

But, if you're a mother, caregiving takes on a whole new meaning. You are bestowed a unique set of responsibilities that come with raising a child. A once peaceful and calm existence becomes a roller coaster ride from hell. Becoming a mother certainly made me grow up fast. And I don't just mean the new gray hairs and wrinkles! The challenge of caring for a new little life while trying to have your own life is like doing the tango. It's like trying to keep your feet from crossing when your brain isn't communicating with your legs. It isn't easy. Like most moms out there, I was constantly juggling a million responsibilities. Trying to raise a family, running a household, and taking care of everyone else was wearing me down to the core. It was an unfamiliar feeling which I didn't like. It seemed for the first time in my adult life, I felt completely out of control. Life was no longer about me. I knew what I needed to do to stay healthy, but finding the time and the motivation to take care of myself just wasn't there. I was so over committed and busy that the last thing on my mind was anything that had to do with me. How would I be able to fit in going to the gym, taking an aerobics class or preparing a nourishing meal, when I barely had time to take a shower?

I like to say I became a "mama-holic." I was addicted to everything related to caring for my child. I remember thinking that it no longer mattered what I wanted or needed. My existence was devoted to doing whatever was needed to make my baby boy's life thrive. The role of mother had consumed every part of me and there was no longer a desire to fulfill my own needs. Ironically, I was actually okay with it. It wasn't until years of being a mama-holic, did my life start to feel incomplete. As my brain fog cleared, I could see there was much more to life than just being a mom. Of course, I loved my child with all my heart, but something else was calling to me. I had forgotten how to be a woman. I had lost *myself.*

I'm going to put myself out on a limb here. One day, around the time my son was approaching middle school, I had a disturbing thought. Something every mother who has been stretched to the limit has had at one time or another. Few would admit to it, but I promise you, most moms have or will feel this way. It didn't happen often, but the first time I had this thought I shuddered. I convinced myself it must mean I was an awful mom. That no mother would, or could, think such a hideous thought. But when that perfect storm came along, and life felt so out of control and overwhelming, it happened. You're probably wondering what this terrible, shocking thought could be? Okay, I'll tell you. I wished I could just run away and leave the kid and husband behind. Not forever, but for a long peaceful weekend away. It was a fleeting thought and didn't last more than a few minutes. But I had it. And I never, ever, thought I would want to spend time away from my child. Remember, I was a mama-holic!

I'll bet many of you moms have thought the same thing at one point. I know you understand exactly how I felt. Feeling ashamed, I silently kept this secret desire to myself. It wasn't like I wished I could abandon my child, but rather I needed to escape the madness of it all for time alone. To just take off the "mama hat" and be a woman. One day I happened to confess my need to get away to a trusted friend. Being a mom herself, I hoped she would understand. Of course, she did. Not only did she understand, she encouraged it! At that moment, I could feel a boulder being lifted off my shoulders. I knew I wasn't a bad mother after all! I was a normal woman with normal needs. It's hard to believe that for years I felt guilty for wanting to spend just a day away. Thank goodness my friend gave me confidence that day. I needed to realize I don't have to go around pretending to be super-mom.

I was fortunate to learn early on how important it is to have a network of moms in your life. If you're a new mother, these women will be your life jacket in a sea of diapers and toys. As your children grow older, these wonderful women may even become your BFF's. I am so grateful for every amazing mom I have met in the many years since my son was born. Having a strong network of moms can serve as a reminder that we are women with feelings, allowed to have moments of regret, doubt and frustration. It's incredibly healthy. Thanks to my wonderful mom friend, I don't feel guilty anymore for wanting to spend a few days alone. Admittedly, it doesn't happen enough, but it will happen again, and I will be a better mom because of it.

What about you? Are you a mama-holic? Do you take time away by yourself? Do you get away for a weekend, a week, or every now and then? It's so important to find YOU time. Being a mother has a lot of responsibility, but you are also a woman with needs. Honor yourself. As a mother, you are making the ultimate sacrifice in life. You are blessed with knowing what it feels like to have unconditional love toward another human being, and at the same time, your patience is being challenged to the very limit. Yes, your children may feel lost without you, but remember how important it is to take some time away to nurture your own soul.

Take a moment to give yourself a pat on the back and a loving hug. Think about how much your own mother sacrificed in her life to raise and care for you. She most likely never had the opportunity or encouragement to take care of herself. Fortunately, in today's world we do. So honor your mother and take some restorative time for you.

The Sandwich Generation

If you're old enough, you may remember the peak of the woman's rights movement. A time when it was acceptable and actually encouraged to delay motherhood and focus on a successful career. Because my parents had adopted my sister and me when they were older, we were never pressured to get married and have kids right away. It gave me the green light to focus on building my career and enjoy traveling the world. Sure, I had often dreamed of having kids someday, but it seemed the timing and partner was never timed right. And with no pressure from society, I didn't worry about it. But by the time I turned 35, the thought of having a baby started finding its way into my mind more and more. I could hear my biological clock ticking loudly and I could feel the pressure to get moving. I suddenly realized the possibility was real that I may never be able to have a child of my own. Then, at age 40, it finally happened. Recently married, a tiny life was growing in my womb. Nine months later, a beautiful and healthy baby boy was born.

These days, it isn't unusual to hear about some celebrity having a baby after age 40. I think it's actually become a trend. What you don't hear is that having a child later in life does have its challenges. For me, it wasn't that I didn't look my age or feel it, because blending in and keeping up with the younger moms was easy. However, there was one big difference. I had parents who were quite a bit older. My mother was 74 and my father 75 when my son was born. While the younger moms could leave their babies with their younger parents, my own parents, being much older, were already dealing with health problems and couldn't offer much help. I would have loved to have my parents babysit for an afternoon, simply so they could experience the joy of being a parent again.

Granted, I'm sure it was pure delight for them just to hold their grandchild, but it didn't give me the satisfaction I was seeking. Unfortunately, this wasn't the only joy they missed. Being older also meant less time left to live in this world, and less time watching their grandchild grow up. It also meant greater challenges for me as well. Never really giving much thought to the possibility of my parents needing my help while raising my own child, I was in for a rude awakening. Sure, I knew my folks were getting older, but I never really stopped to think of what would happen if they couldn't take care of themselves. I had been living in denial for too long. Because that's what kids do. No matter how old our parents become, we still want to turn to them when life gets difficult. I expected my parents to be that pillar of support to the very end and it was a frightening thought to imagine they could no longer take care of me. But it happened. And it came at a time when I needed them too.

As a new mom trying to figure it all out, I longed to share this experience with my mother. But, by the time my son was born, my mother was already starting to lose her mental function. She was often forgetful and confused, and her health was declining quickly. I watched as our roles began to shift. I found her needing my help more than I did hers. My father, who was a lifelong smoker, wasn't in much better health. His fifty year tobacco habit had finally taken a toll on his health and he was no longer able handle the errands and household chores. As their phone calls for help became more frequent, it became very clear I needed to be there for them. And while this shift was happening, my life was also consumed with a new baby at home. Feeling torn, I was caught right smack dab in the middle of two generations. I had fallen into what is known as the "sandwich generation." The generation when you have older parents who need your care while raising your own children at the same time. With many women putting off motherhood until their late 30s and early 40s, I see this becoming more common. I actually have friends in this very same situation. They find themselves torn between being the loyal daughter and being the responsible mother. It's a difficult balancing act. You are trying to meet the needs of everyone. Unless you happen to be one of those older wealthy celebrity moms who can hire all the extra hands needed, you will fall into the 99% of us who end up tired, stressed, and anxious.

After years of bouncing back and forth between the role of responsible daughter and overwhelmed new mother, I decided to take a break from the madness. I planned a family weekend getaway to a safari adventure park about an hour away. The stress of running around day and night caring for my parents had taken up so much of my time that I had forgotten how to have fun with my own family. It was my birthday, yet making the decision to go away at a time when both of my parents were at two separate nursing homes was very difficult. Easing my fears, my husband reminded me it wasn't too far in case of an emergency. So we packed up the car and headed out. But low and behold, an emergency did happen. We hadn't even driven half way to our destination, when my cell phone rang. It was the nursing home where my dad was staying. He had tried to get up and fallen, and they wanted to know what to do. Like a scene out of a soap opera, as I was on the phone talking with my father's nursing home, my other phone line rang. Hesitant to pick it up, I answered. It was the lead nurse at the nursing home where my mother resided. She had fallen down too. You can only imagine the stress and anxiety I was feeling at that very moment. I couldn't believe my luck.

Actually, incidents like this happened all the time. My parents were confused, ill, and stubborn. Hospital visits, emergency rooms, and nursing homes were just a normal part of my existence. After making sure their falls weren't life threatening, I calmly told each person to call 911 and report back to me from the hospital. There was simply nothing more I could do. As I ended each call, I could feel the guilt building up inside me. I felt as if I was being a horrible daughter. How could I just leave them alone like that? But my inner voice told me if I didn't take this time away, I would most definitely have a serious mental breakdown. Taking those two days away were as necessary to me as breathing. I needed it. Having fun that weekend took some effort, but I was able to enjoy the time away with my husband and son. I may not have slept well that night, but the simple act of allowing myself time away from the daily worry and stress, gave my mind a much needed rest.

If you happen to be a woman caught in the "sandwich generation" and feeling overwhelmed, I hope you will take advice from me and find time to care for yourself. If you happen to have elderly parents that live far away, the stress is still there. The challenges may be different, but the guilt, worry and grief are the same. You may not be faced with the same daily challenges, but you may end up with more guilt. I have always felt grateful that I had the gift of caring for my parents until the end of their lives. Sure, the stress almost landed me in the hospital, but the peace I feel inside knowing I was there in their time of need will stay with me forever. Everyone will cope with aging parents in a different way. No one way is perfect. You have to do what makes your heart feel good, but take care to not neglect your needs in the process. I still remember something that our estate lawyer said when we were preparing the power of attorney for my mom. He said that in his many years of practice, he often saw the caregiver's spouse die first, as a result of all the stress from caring for their loved one. Ironically, my father died two months before my mother, even though she was the one in worse health.

When you reach this point, or if you're already there, it's critical to take time for you. Use the exercises in this book to nurture yourself every day. Make sure to eat nourishing food and find ways to move your body every day. I don't have an answer for how to make the situation go away. It's a part of your life experience. But what I *can* give you is hope, guidance, and encouragement that someday it will be normal again. The most important thing you can do is take care of your own health. Because if you aren't healthy, you won't be able to care for anyone, even your loved ones. I know it isn't always easy to do, but if you make your health a priority you will feel better and have more energy to care for those who are most important to you. And that may mean sometimes you just have to say "no" and not feel guilty.

Don't be afraid to ask for help, hire a caregiver, or discuss options for assisted living facilities. And above all, act from your heart. The decisions we must make when our parents reach their end stage of life is emotionally exhausting. We wish we didn't have to acknowledge their mortality, but by doing so, we are honoring their life. But also remember that you are important too. While I was caring for my parents and also caring for my baby boy, I nearly forgot about myself.

10 Steps to Survive Being a Caregiver

1. Take at least 10 minutes each day to do something nice for yourself. Whether it's just 10 minutes of massaging your feet or 10 minutes of sitting outside in the sun. Do anything that makes you feel good.

2. Ask your spouse to take on more of the parenting responsibility while you care for your parent. Having one less thing to worry about will make a huge difference in your stress level.

3. Hire a part-time or live-in caregiver for your loved one. Don't feel as if you are the only person who can handle the daily care. Even if your parent is resistant to having a stranger in the house, you need the relief.

4. Hire a cleaning person and/or someone to help prepare meals. These are simple jobs that you can hand over to

someone else, and it will make your life much easier.

5. Eat a healthy diet and avoid alcohol. Chronic stress and anxiety will definitely cause you to crave sugary snacks and junk food. Resist the temptation to eat on the run or consume stimulants like sugar, alcohol and caffeine. Eating healthy food means a clearer mind and more energy.

6. Get daily exercise. If you don't have time for the gym, simply take a 20 minute walk around the block. Exercise is so important for managing your stress and taming tension. When I had no control over the craziness of my life, I made sure to take brisk walks every day.

7. Set boundaries and stick to them. Don't over-schedule your day. There will be times when you need to say no. It's okay, you have needs too. Explore outside resources for help. There are many organizations that provide assistance like transportation for the elderly and disabled.

8. Take a yoga, qi gong, tai chi or other mind-body class at least once a week. A wonderful way to ground yourself, release tension, balance your mind and lower cortisol.

9. Once or twice a week do something fun! Don't forget the importance of letting go and having a good time. You can go see a funny film, visit an amusement park, ride bikes, play at the beach, throw a party, or have dinner with good friends. Do anything that makes you smile.

10. Remember to breathe. Take nice deep cleansing breaths several times a day. Your brain needs plenty of oxygen to stay alert, think clearly and function optimally.

Chapter 4
Stress... the Other Deadly Six Letter Word

The body is an amazing machine. It is designed to survive. It seems we can abuse it over and over when we are younger and it just bounces back. But in truth, the body is coping. It is doing what is was created to do, stay alive. Through a process called allostasis, our body is always striving for balance. When something upsets our nervous system, we are driven to find relief. Think about it. If you are feeling cold, you put on a jacket, if you are hungry, you eat food, if you are tired, you (want) to take a nap. This is how the body copes. But what happens if we don't listen to our signals? What if we rely on caffeine for energy, skip meals because we are too busy to eat or simply ignore our natural instincts. How many of us busy women are walking around feeling stressed and overwhelmed, never taking time to care for our needs? A lot. Eventually, we find ourselves in *allostatic load*, when the wear and tear on the body grows over time through repeated exposed chronic stress, causing our body to wear out.

You may wonder how stress harms the body. When we perceive any kind of threat, our bodies go into a stress response, what is commonly known as fight-or-flight. Our sympathetic nervous system (SNS), kicks in and prepares the body to run away from danger or be ready for battle. Without this mechanism our species would have died out a long time ago. When our sympathetic nervous system (SNS) is activated our body starts to produce adrenaline. Adrenaline is our short-term stress hormone which increases our heart rate, blood pressure, shuts down digestion and directs glucose into our blood stream for quick energy. We need adrenaline to give us the ability to get out of danger's way. In the early years of human existence, this was our built in survival mechanism. If you were being chased by a saber toothed cat, you needed every ounce of energy to run away and hide. However, in today's world we seem to be running away from "saber toothed cats" all the time. Of course, not literally, but the body can't distinguish the difference. And we certainly don't need adrenaline pumping out all day, seven days a week.

Yet, that's exactly what happens when we are rushing around every day trying to please everyone and putting out fires. You may be thinking, but I'm not always rushing around. Still, while you may not be physically running around, your brain doesn't separate out anxious thoughts and physical stress. In your everyday life, you may not be chased by lions or fighting off unfriendly neighbors (hopefully not), but your brain doesn't know the difference. Whenever you feel worried, hurried, frazzled, or stressed, you are causing your body to go into a fight-or-flight response. Your thoughts are sending signals that danger is near. Your body reacts the same way when you are rushing to your next appointment or to pick up the kids, just as it would if you were being chased by a saber tooth cat.

Just think of how many times a day you are rushing around, trying to accomplish a million tasks and taking care of everyone but yourself. In today's world, we are constantly overwhelmed with outside stimulation, whether it's the 500 email messages in your inbox, the evening news filled with violence, or social media which never allows our mind to rest. It's no wonder we feel stressed out all the time! We have more reasons to feel stressed today that we ever did in history. Imagine what this can do to your health over a long period of time.

When we constantly produce adrenaline, over time our bodies begin to have higher cortisol levels. Cortisol is our long-term stress hormone and our body's survival mechanism in times of famine, flood, or when food is scarce. It does a great job of storing energy and slowing down metabolism. In fact, cortisol works so well to preserve energy, that it causes you to store the fat around your waist. Which ends up as that dreaded muffin top. Ready to de-stress yet? Consider these other health issues that come along with living an over-stressed life. You will be on the fast track to weight gain, poor skin, chronic fatigue, migraines, elevated blood pressure and even high blood sugar. Chronically high cortisol can eventually lead to adrenal fatigue, which then leads to lower levels of cortisol. When you reach this point you will be exhausted all the time and feel awful. Your body will no longer produce enough cortisol to give you energy, and you'll have what's known as adrenal burnout.

Dr. Sara Gottfried, author of "The Hormone Cure" calls the stress response "tend and befriend," in women, because we seem to react differently than men when it comes to stress. According to Dr. Sara, women tend to seek out the company of other women and talk through issues, while men typically withdraw and/or lash out. It used to be the belief that women and men produced the same amount of cortisol in response to stress. We now know that women actually produce more oxytocin, which is the hormone responsible for the feelings of bonding, which would explain why we are more likely to turn to each other in times of stress rather than suffer alone in silence. This is great for women, but not so good for men!

Is Stress Making You Sick?

I hope you don't need a doctor to convince you that stress is harming your health. Plenty of studies have shown that chronic stress is linked to heart disease, type 2 diabetes, inflammatory disease, weakened immunity, cancer, and even thyroid function.

There is no magic pill for treating stress because it's not an actual disease. However, we can't escape stress entirely. It's a part of being alive in this day and age. But, if you let your stress take over, eventually it will most likely lead to serious disease. You see, when your body is under stress, it's in distress, or as I like to say, in a state of "dis-ease." I'm convinced that chronic stress lead to the development of my thyroid nodule. All those years of burning the candle at both ends took a toll on my adrenal function, most likely affecting my thyroid from producing enough hormone. And when that happens, the thyroid slows down and we end up with symptoms like cold hands, cold feet, hair loss and foggy brain. Sound familiar? It's not surprising that so many women are walking around today with underactive or overactive thyroids.

So, how do you get your stress under control? You must look honestly at your life and get to the root of your triggers. Instead of waiting for your health to decline, it's better to take action to remove the parts of your life causing you stress. Yes, I realize it's easier said than done. But that is why you are reading this book! To learn ways to eliminate stress, bring more joy into your life and find time to relax. If you are one of the 1 in 5 women in this country taking antidepressants, I hope you will pay special attention to the section on yoga and meditation. Especially since antidepressants are now the most overly prescribed drugs in this country. Unfortunately, women are more likely to be prescribed a medication for symptoms that can usually be treated with diet and lifestyle changes. I know, because I was one of those stressed out women prescribed anxiety pills. Determined to not become dependent on a pill, I was able to overcome my anxiety naturally and I know other women can too. If you have been diagnosed with depression or anxiety, I encourage a discussion with your doctor about options other than lifelong medication. Many women have experienced great results from using alternative therapies and holistic healers such as acupuncture, biofeedback, psychotherapy, nutrition counseling, or working with naturopathic doctors.

When my life was spiraling out of control, my blood pressure started creeping up and I suffered from heart palpitations. I woke up every morning with a headache, no energy and feeling awful. Having never experienced such sickness before, I knew something was terribly wrong. I had body aches and pains and felt tired all the time. I had very little energy. Like most busy women, I turned to caffeine and found myself craving daily Starbucks vanilla lattés. Of course, it didn't help. It only made me feel worse. The caffeine caused my adrenaline to soar and the sugar spiked my glucose. And when my blood sugar came crashing down, it left me feeling even more tired. After several months of my new Starbucks habit, that classic afternoon slump started to hit me real bad. Every day at around 2pm, I would feel so exhausted that all I could do was stretch across the sofa and wonder what was happening to me. It was a weird feeling. My body felt tired, but my brain was still wired. I wanted to sleep, but I wasn't sleepy. It was a strange place to be.

My life was moving at light speed and there were many days when it seemed impossible to take a moment to breathe. I just kept going and going. Juggling a million tasks and taking on even more if anyone asked, I was caught in a vortex of "to do's." If my son's school needed volunteers, I was there, if my mother or father needed a ride to the doctor, I was there, if the dog or cat needed to go to the vet, I was there. The list went on and on. I just couldn't say no to anyone! And still, I knew I was handling too much, worrying about too many people, and feeling unhappy in my life. One particular day, something happened to help me realize that it was time to slow down. I was visiting my father at the hospital thirty minutes away from home. I had driven there during lunch after a busy morning of phone calls with family and doctors. While I was there, my cell phone rang and it was my son's school. Worried something terrible had happened I answered it right way. It was the school secretary calling because my son had somehow ripped a hole in his pants that stretched from his knee all the way to below his crotch. She called to ask if

I could bring him a new pair of pants. I thought about it for a minute, I could rush home now, pick up pants, rush to school, drop them off and then turn around in less than an hour to pick him up. Or, I could stay at the hospital and let my son spend the remainder of the day exposing part of his leg. As I glanced down at my father lying in his hospital bed, I realized that every day with him could be my last. So, I told the secretary to let my son wear his torn jeans for the rest of the school day and I wasn't coming. And I'm glad I did. That hour with my father was precious, as he died only weeks later. And when I picked up my son from school, his pants were "mended" by the school secretary with about a dozen safety pins. All was good.

That day I learned to not sweat the small stuff. Torn jeans were not the end of the world. There will always be something to stress about. We need to save our energy for more important worries like a sick child or ailing parent, and let go of the smaller things we can't control. If you take a moment and think about everything that stressed you out today, would any of your worries cause the world to end? Don't be the person who stresses about the weather, or if your child will make it onto the soccer team. Life is too short to sweat the small stuff. Relax, breathe and all will be fine. Your first step to eliminate stress is to take a serious look at what may be causing you stress in your life. Then make a plan for change. Whether it be a toxic relationship, stressful work environment, over-booked schedule, out of control kids, or an unsatisfying home life, you must look honestly at your life. Do you eat junk food when you are feeling stressed? Do you turn to alcohol to unwind at the end of the day? What can you do each day to move toward a happier and healthier tomorrow? Use the meditation exercise to visualize the life you want to live. Set an intention to reduce your stress by making small changes every day. Perhaps you can keep a journal and reflect on your progress. There are many things you can do to start bringing more positivity into your life. When you think more positive thoughts, your stress starts to melt away.

10 Ways to Reduce Stress

1. **Take a deep breath**. Breathing deeply activates the para-sympathetic nervous system, the response that counteracts our fight-or-flight mode. Start by breathing in slowly through your nose, counting to five, then exhaling through your mouth to a count of five.

2. **Meditate.** Sit quietly and close your eyes. Let your thoughts float by and bring attention to your breath. Even a five minute meditation will rejuvenate your mind.

3. **Keep a gratitude journal.** Using a journal or notebook, write down five things you are grateful for at the end of each day. We tend to focus on the things that cause us stress, but by reflecting on the gifts in life, we are encouraged to feel happier and more loving.

4. **Eat dark chocolate**. Chocolate lovers, rejoice! Dark chocolate is heart healthy and a yummy antioxidant. It also stimulates the feel good receptors in the brain. Look for at least 70% cacao and savor only about an ounce a day.

5. **Get a massage**. Schedule a monthly therapeutic massage to calm your nervous system. Human touch is healing to the body and stimulates the hormone oxytocin. Even a massage once every few months will calm your nervous system.

6. **Soak in a tub with Epsom salts**. Pour a cup of Epsom salts into warm bath water and add 2-3 drops of lavender essential oil. The magnesium in the Epsom salts relaxes your central nervous system and will even help you sleep better.

7. **Think positive thoughts**. The more you think positive, the happier you will feel. Try to see things as the glass being half full, rather than half empty. By focusing on the positive things in your life you can retrain your brain to bring more joy into your life.

8. **Diffuse essential oils**. Lavender is my favorite essential oil. It's calming, healing, and reduces stress. Other wonderful oils for calming are doTERRA's Serenity and Balance blends, or Peppermint, Grapefruit and Lemon. You can place a few drops into a diffuser or in a bowl of warm water and inhale.

9. **Meet a friend for tea**. A wonderful way to de-stress! Remember the "tend and befriend" response. Talking with a friend lowers cortisol and raises our feel good hormones. Try sipping herbal teas like Chamomile and Holy Basil for ultimate relaxation.

10. **Go for a walk in nature**. Just the simple act of being in nature lowers our blood pressure and heart rate. When you are feeling especially stressed, taking a walk is a great way to calm down. If you're stuck inside, try looking out a window with views of flowers or trees, upload a beautiful nature scene as your screensaver or watch a nature video on Youtube.com.

It's all About the Breath

Ready to learn a quick way to calm down? Take a deep breath. Sounds too simple doesn't it? But when you take a deep breath, you start to activate your parasympathetic nervous system. It's the opposite of your fight-or-flight response, the PNS is responsible for calming down your nervous system. When you breathe slowly and deeply, it signals your brain that the danger has passed. Your heart rate slows, your blood pressure drops and normal digestion resumes. Your body enters a state of calm. Isn't that wonderful?

It took me many years to figure this out. As a child, I took weekly ballet lessons. I remember the private studio, located in the teacher's flat on the second floor. She lived in an affluent old San Francisco neighborhood; an artsy woman with graying hair. At the end of every class, she would have all of us little girls sit in a circle and do these strange exercises. She would have us stick out our tongues and try to make them touch our chins. Then she had us lie on our backs and breathe. We were instructed to watch our bellies go up and down. As a six-year-old girl, it was a lot of fun. She would then end our class with a ceremony of throwing some "magic dust" into the fireplace, and the embers would turn all kinds of pretty colors.

I didn't know it then, but what my ballet teacher was doing was teaching us to be mindful. Something that we all naturally are born to do. If you ever watch a very young child breathe, you will see their bellies rise and fall with each breath. We are born to breathe using our entire diaphragm; it's not until we grow up that we forget. As we age and experience the stresses of life, we begin to breathe shallow and faster. It's a natural stress response that we don't even notice. While you are out and about one day, stop and pay attention to your breathing for a moment. Is it slow and deep? Are you taking full breaths, so that your belly rises and falls? Or are you breathing quick and shallow? Try taking a deep breath and see what happens.

Breathing is the most important bodily function we have. It's a part of our autonomic nervous system. Those automatic functions that keep us alive, like blood pressure, heart rate, digestion, and sweating. It happens automatically; we don't have to think about it. Yet, we often breathe incorrectly. We manage to take in enough oxygen to stay alive, but are we taking in enough oxygen to *thrive*? Consider this, deep breathing reduces stress.

When you breathe deeply, your diaphragm fills with oxygen and you stimulate the vagus nerve. Which is the main nerve responsible for taking us out of the stress response. If you ever wonder why you feel tired in the middle of day for no reason, it could very well be that you have been breathing shallow all day and your brain doesn't have enough oxygen.

Belly Breathing

Most of us only use the top half of our lungs to breathe. So we really don't take in enough oxygen to nourish all the cells in our bodies. It's important for us to learn how to breathe correctly, using our entire diaphragm. Practice the steps below to learn how to utilize and fill your entire lungs with life-giving oxygen.

- ♥ Lie on your back or sit upright in a chair. Take a slow, deep breath to the count of four, watching to see when your belly begin to rise.
- ♥ Pause for a moment.
- ♥ Breathe out slowly to a count of five. When you get to the end of your exhale, force out the last remaining air.
- ♥ Breathe in slowly again for a count of four.
- ♥ Repeat this sequence for at least seven rounds of deep breaths.

Congratulations, you have successfully put yourself in relaxation mode.

"Be there for others, but never leave yourself behind."
— Dodinsky

Chapter 5
Say Goodbye to Anxiety

I have had a life-long struggle with anxiety. I'm not unique, many women experience anxiety yet are embarrassed and ashamed to talk about it. In fact, millions of people in this country suffer with anxiety every day. We try to hide our insecurities, our phobias, and pretend that nothing bothers us beyond the "normal" worries. Many of us are walking around and silently suffering from our fears. If you are one of those anxiety ridden people, I hope you will not feel alone anymore. By sharing my story, I want to give you the confidence to make changes. And if you are lucky enough to not suffer from anxiety, then hopefully you will take what you learn and share with a friend.

While we are quick to complain about being stressed out and having too much to do, how many times do you hear your friends tell you they had a panic attack, or were so anxious they couldn't even drive to the grocery store? Probably not often. But I guarantee you have friends in your life right now who are secretly hiding their anxiety and fears. Maybe it's you. Well, please take comfort and know that you are not alone. Let me show you how to quiet your mind, confront your fears and say goodbye to anxiety. It may take some time and patience, but the reward is so worth it.

First, let me explain the difference between stress and anxiety. Although they often go hand in hand, there is a big difference. When we are frequently stressed, it can lead to anxiety.

So, understanding how to deal with stress is very important in healing from anxiety. As we learned in Chapter 4, chronic stress affects our central nervous system; it encourages us to eat unhealthy food, not get enough sleep, drink too much coffee and make poor health choices. And when the body is working hard to overcome the effects of stress, the perfect conditions are set for anxiety to take over. A hormonal imbalance can also lead to anxiety, especially when we don't produce enough oxytocin and serotonin, our feel good hormones. And chronic stress is a major cause of hormonal imbalance. If we don't manage our stress, we won't be able to overcome our anxiety. Let me also point out that both stress and anxiety begin in the brain. They both are created by our thoughts. Stress is a result of our mind being overloaded with responsibilities, like work, kids, school, errands, relationships, and never enough time; while anxiety develops from fearing the unknown, having phobias, excessive worry, or feeling like something bad will happen for no apparent reason.

I will never forget the night I had my first panic attack. I was only 14 and had no idea why I felt like I was going to die. It was in the evening and I was getting ready for bed. Suddenly, this overwhelming feeling of impending doom and fear came over me. I didn't know what was happening and it was very frightening. At the time, my mother had a business at home and was working late as usual. I went into her office and said I didn't feel well. I couldn't explain why, only that I felt like I was going to die. My body was trembling, my heart racing and my mind in a panic.

My aunt, who is my mother's sister, lived with us at the time. She was the calm and easy going person in the family. Not wanting my mother to panic herself, she took me back to my bedroom, told me to lie on my stomach and put my rear end in the air. She said it was probably trapped gas and this awkward position will help move it out. I can laugh about it now, but the fear I was experiencing at the time was no joke. Yet, that simple act of redirecting my thoughts to my butt sticking up in the air made the panic attack go away. Seriously. Of course, I wasn't suffering from gas, my stomach didn't even hurt. But taking my mind off the panic attack and into another thought pattern was apparently the right thing to do. I just didn't realize it back then.

Fortunately, I didn't have another panic attack until a decade later. Although, I still experienced anxious thoughts about certain situations. Throughout my twenties and into my thirties, I would have occasional panic attacks, but they would pass quickly and I could go on with a normal life. However, nothing compared to the anxiety I experienced after age 40. Around the time of my parent's death, my anxiety had become so bad that it was taking away all my enjoyment of life. It had become so serious that I often worried I may die of a heart attack, even though I didn't have heart disease. In my head I knew it wasn't logical, but the anxiety kept my mind racing with crazy thoughts. This is how anxiety takes control of your life. Your thoughts go wild and take you into a world of "what ifs." What if I die; who will raise my child? What if I pass out on the freeway; will I crash? What if I have cancer? What if this pain in my leg is a blood clot? What if I can't breathe? And on and on!

One day, as I stood in the kitchen, watching my husband walk out the door on his way to work, I could feel my anxiety coming on. In an instant, thoughts of impending doom tried to take over my mind. But this time, I resisted. Standing there trembling, panic stricken and feeling fearful that I might pass out, I closed my eyes and imagined my sweet little boy, and how I promised him mommy will always be there to watch him grow up. I started to shift my anxious thoughts to those of love for my son. How could I not take care of myself and risk the possibility of leaving him motherless? It was time to do something soon, I couldn't live the rest of my life feeling this fear. At that moment, I knew it was either do or die. Either I take action and make a change, or I continue to live in fear and misery, missing out on all the joys in life.

Let it Flow

Healing from anxiety was one of the most empowering health changes that I have made. If you suffer from anxiety then you understand what I mean. To no longer be controlled by your fears is like lifting a piano off your chest. You can breathe, you can do things without fear, and you can live freely again. It was the journey away from my anxious thoughts that saved my sanity and gave me new life. I hear about too many women who suffer from anxiety and turn to pills. But medication doesn't have to be the answer. I overcame my anxiety without taking drugs. It wasn't easy, because healing naturally takes time and patience, but eventually, I was able to retrain my brain to more positive and calming thoughts.

My very Zen-like sister taught me an important lesson about letting go. Growing up together, she knew how I worried about every little thing. Even though she was my younger sister, I always turned to her when my fears were spiraling out of control. Unlike me, she never seemed to worry much or suffer from phobias. She was the one I counted on when my nervous system needed a rest. One evening, around the time our parents died, I felt myself going into a major panic attack. It was late at night and my young son was sleeping upstairs. Alone, with no one around, I called my sister. This time, rather than the usual calming me down session, she told me to refocus my thoughts. She asked me if what I was worrying about would change by continuing to worry. No, it would not. She asked if I having a rational thought? No, I was not. It was then that I realized my irrational thought pattern had been controlling my mind to the point where I could no longer control my thoughts.

Have you ever heard the saying "let it flow?" It's based on an ancient Chinese Taoist saying and very wise words indeed. If you spent all your time worrying about this and that, not only would the situation have the same outcome, but you would end up wasting precious time. Imagine what wonderful thoughts you could be enjoying rather than worrying about things you can't control. I get it. I was once a chronic worrier. I had convinced myself that it would never change, that being a worry wart was part of who I was. Hey, it even runs in my family! But let me be the first to tell you, you can change your worrisome thoughts. You can retrain that wonderful brain of yours to start thinking lovely, happy, and productive thoughts.

How do you do this? Well, when you find yourself worrying about anything, turn your attention to the present moment. For example, let's say you are at home and start worrying about your child on their first day of school. Your thoughts start spiraling out of control. You imagine that your son fell off the monkey bars, hit his head and will have permanent brain damage, or your daughter wandered off campus and a stranger coaxed her into a car. Yes, seems pretty far-fetched, but if you're a chronic worrier, your thoughts can get out of control pretty fast. So, when you notice your worrisome thoughts, begin to direct your attention to something in the present moment, like an object in the room. Look around you, what do you see? Focus on the colors of your surroundings. What do you hear? Listen to the sounds of your environment. Maybe look out the window. Admire the trees, look down the street, peak into the cars that drive by. The goal of this exercise is to distract your worrisome thoughts back to the present. At first, it may seem difficult. You may find yourself bouncing back between your present thoughts and what you are worried about, and that is perfectly normal. In time, it will become more natural to change your thoughts and bring them back to the present.

According to Dr. Rick Hanson, a neuropsychologist and meditation teacher, we can actually rewire our brains to cultivate positive emotions, inner peace and lasting happiness. In his book "Buddha's Brain: The Practical Neuroscience of Happiness, Love, and Wisdom" he explores how changing our thoughts can literally change the structure of our brain. Through the process of neuroplasticity, our brain is continually changing its shape and structure. Dr. Hanson points out that the more the mind has negative thoughts, like self-criticism or being angry at someone, the more our brain will gradually take the shape of the worse mood and be less resilient. Therefore, being upset makes us more prone to getting upset more often.

This also means that we have the ability to shape our brain to induce a happier mood. If we routinely focus our thoughts on the positive things around us, like the beauty of nature, the sounds of kids playing, or the freshness of the morning air, our brain will start to take on a shape that has greater resilience. We then encourage a more positive mood, positive emotion and deepen our insight. Think of it as physical exercise for your brain. Just like your muscles get stronger and can hold heavier objects, your brain is getting stronger and able to think more positive thoughts with more practice. It's amazing to learn about this discovery of the human brain. As it gives us the power to be able to shape our own thoughts.

Meditation

Meditation is another very effective way to reduce anxiety and stress. It has been shown to reduce blood pressure, help with depression, increase memory function, and calm anxiety. It brings mental clarity and focus, and can be useful in dealing with stress. When we meditate, we are releasing external distractions and turning our attention inward, being present in our own bodies. When I first tried meditation, it was difficult for me to sit still. My mind kept wandering and my breathing was shallow. It just didn't feel natural to me, but I kept trying, and eventually I could settle into my breath. It was wonderful to enjoy the stillness. For me, it was easier to start with guided meditations. I found it hard to just sit quietly in silence. My meditations usually involve visualizing a beautiful place in nature, a place that makes me feel safe and calm. Often, my imagined places change, but the feeling of peace and serenity remain the same.

If you've never tried to meditate, maybe it's time. As a busy, stressed out woman, it is a wonderful way to slow down and quiet your mind. Meditation has a wealth of health benefits, from improving memory to reducing your risk of heart disease. If you're like me and not comfortable sitting quietly at first, a good way to start is by trying guided meditations. My favorite meditations are offered free online by Deepak Chopra and Oprah Winfrey, or you can find your own favorites on youtube.com. Some wellness centers and adult schools offer meditation classes as well. Or, you can simply close your eyes for 10 minutes and sit comfortably, focusing on your breath or repeating a mantra. If privacy is a challenge, you can also put your hands on your heart, close your eyes and listen to your own heartbeat for a few minutes.

The goal of meditation is to do something mindful in order to quiet the part of your brain which is always thinking. Not only does meditation lower your stress, but it also does wonders to reduce anxiety. So, are you ready to give it a try!

Simple Meditation for Relaxation

1. Sit quietly in a comfortable position.
2. Close your eyes.
3. Begin to relax your muscles, starting at your feet and moving all the way up to your face.
4. Breathing through your nose, repeat a calming word such as "peace" silently to yourself. Breathe slowly and naturally.
5. Do this for 10 to 15 minutes.
6. If you find your mind being distracted by a sound or random thoughts, just bring your thoughts back to the word "peace" and continue.

You don't always have to sit still in order to quiet your mind. Moving meditation is another form of mindfulness, taking your thoughts away from your internal chatter and bringing it back into the present moment. When you focus on your breath for instance, your mind can't focus on random thoughts at the same time. Being fully present takes practice, but in time you can learn to turn off your internal chatter and quiet the mind.

Moving Meditations

- ♥ Take a yoga class and focus on your breath
- ♥ Put on your favorite song and move to the music
- ♥ Go for a walk and be present to every sight and sound
- ♥ Dance slowly with another person and feel their heartbeat
- ♥ Watch your child sleep
- ♥ Attend a meditation circle or a drum circle

Om, My Yoga

I am in love with yoga. I can say with all honestly that yoga gave me new life. After all the stress that I had endured while my parents were sick, my body felt like it was falling apart. I was plagued with anxiety and frequent panic attacks and searched for something to calm my mind and bring peace back into my life. Yoga was my answer. I had no idea that yoga would change my life in such a powerful way.

Yoga is many things to different people, and to me it was about healing. I remember walking into my first yoga class and feeling a little awkward. After finding a space in the back of the room, I rolled out my brand new mat and removed my shoes. At first the poses looked intimidating and the pace of the class felt too fast. It was a challenge to keep up with the other students. When the teacher instructed us to focus on the breath, I felt like I was going to hyperventilate. Yet, the whole experience left me feeling calm like never before. I loved the feeling; it was something I needed so desperately, and I wanted it to stay with me all day.

I began to try different yoga classes and different teachers. Each one had his/her own particular style and energy. Some were great and others left me feeling just okay. But the practice of yoga introduced me to a body and mind connection I had never felt before. It was after going to regular yoga classes that my anxiety began to happen less and less often. Every class I took gave me one more reason to love yoga. But it was a particular teacher that really made the biggest difference, someone who opened my heart to reconnecting with the inner self. Her name was Bette, a soft spoken woman who brought a peaceful calm to each class. It was through her gentle manner and positive energy that I began to feel real change. As she guided us through the asanas (yoga poses), I could feel my body releasing past emotions. While opening up my heart center and hips, trapped emotions were being set free. I would be holding a pose and suddenly, these flashbacks of various moments in my life entered my mind.

At the end of one particular class, we were lying in savasana (relaxation pose) and Bette asked us to think back to when we were a child. She told us to feel the security and warmth of our mother's love. Having recently lost my mother, it was an intensely emotional moment. Tears rolled down my face while I lay there on my mat, missing my mother and feeling her warmth and love. I learned at that moment how to fill myself with love whenever I chose. It is always inside of me. It's always inside all of us. We choose to embrace or ignore the positive emotions in our minds. Because if we change our thoughts, we change our mood. We hold the power to create our own happiness. Feelings of peace and love are never farther than our own minds.

When people think of yoga, they imagine bodies twisted up in unnatural positions and being covered in tight fitting clothing. But yoga is so much deeper than yoga pants and downward facing dog. It's an incredible tool to keep your prana (life force) flowing and to clear trapped emotional trauma. In the yogic tradition, it is believed that two reasons exist for people remaining stuck in negative emotions. The first is samskaras, or karmic knots, that develop in response to each trauma or loss. Performing asanas while focusing on the breath helps release these karmic knots, freeing emotions and the related tension in our body. The second is a lack of prana, or vital life force, in the system. When our prana is low because of stress, overwork, or simply being too busy, we tend to feel sluggish. Practicing yoga with attention to the breath expands the lungs, bringing in more oxygen, creating a state of mental alertness, and calming the body.

Of all the methods I used to overcome my stress and anxiety, there is no better one I can recommend than to practice yoga. If you're not in the best physical shape right now, try not to be intimidated by the poses. There are so many different styles and classes to choose from. Start with a beginner class if it's your first time and take it slow. In time, your body will cooperate more and you will amaze yourself. Remember, yoga is not only about the poses, it's about the breath. When practicing, always concentrate on your breath and only move as deeply as you feel comfortable. Honor your body and listen to its clues. Yoga should not hurt! If you make a commitment to practice yoga at least once a week, it will make a huge difference in your life. Trust me.

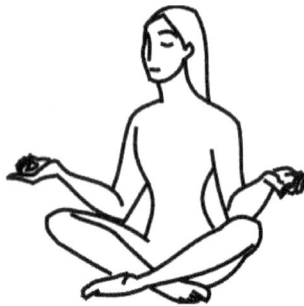

Relaxation comes from letting go of tense thoughts.
— Frances Wilshire

PART TWO
Nourish Your Body

"If we didn't eat junk, we would have this wisdom inside of our body that actually tells us what it needs."

- Donna Gates

Chapter 6
Eat Real Food

If you met me today, you would never guess that at one time I lived on a diet of pizza, bagels, muffins and pasta. And when I was a teenager, I even ate Taco Bell and loved Doritos nacho cheese tortilla chips with a Milky Way candy bar. Yep, I wasn't that different from everyone else. Granted, I've never been more than ten pounds overweight, but that doesn't mean I didn't struggle with my body image. For years, I used to exercise five days a week just to be able to go out for breakfast and dessert with my girlfriends. We would fill up on pancakes, muffins and pasta and often just ordered dessert. Believe it or not, I used to think that because I wasn't eating any fat, and only loading up on carbs, that I was being healthy. If only I knew! It wasn't until I changed the foods I ate that my weight finally stopped going up and down. As I started to eat more vegetables, healthy fats and less sugar, my cravings started to go away. The added bonus was that I ended up with better digestion and glowing skin.

Changing the way I ate also opened the door to incredible changes in my energy and mind. After making the decision to heal my body, the first thing I set out to do was to eat healthier food. All my life I had thought that I was a healthy eater; avoiding butter, red meat, pork, fried foods, chicken skin, fast food, avocado, cream cheese, nuts and coconut oil. I thought I was doing everything right, until I studied nutrition and learned the truth. I was doing some things right, like avoiding fatty meats, fried foods, fast food and processed food. But I also realized I wasn't eating nearly enough vegetables and healthy fat. As I started to fill my plate with an abundance of raw and cooked vegetables, only then did I start to feel a huge shift in my energy and mood. After living with years of frequent brain fog, it was like someone cleaned the glass and life became so much clearer. My memory improved and it was no longer a struggle to stay focused. I woke up each morning with energy that I hadn't experienced in over a decade. I was amazed that by simply adding in more vegetables and healthy fat that it could make such a huge difference on the way I felt. But it did!

Okay, so filling half your plate with vegetables is a smart and healthy change to your diet. How would you like to know another small, but powerful change you can do to help you lose weight, ditch cravings and start to glow. It's very simple, give up processed foods. These packaged "foods" are high in sodium, loaded with sugar, are calorie dense, and have chemicals in them you can't even pronounce. Processed foods are the number one reason people gain weight, feel lousy, and can't lose their belly fat. When I tell people to stop eating processed foods, they immediately think of cookies, chips and candy. But oh, there is so much more. Did you know that breakfast cereal is one of the most highly processed foods? Yep, and so is wheat bread, lunch meat, whole grain crackers, frozen meals (even healthy ones) and canned soup. Actually, processed food is anything that comes from a plant, and I'm not talking about the kind of plant that grows in the ground.

Here's an easy way to determine if your favorite foods are processed.

- ✓ Does it come in a box, plastic wrapper, or can?
- ✓ Does it list ingredients on the label that you don't recognize or can't pronounce?

✓ Can you store it on your shelf for more than a month without spoiling?

✓ Would your great grandmother not have a clue what it is?

If you can answer yes to even one of those questions, I'm sorry to say, it is probably a processed food.

If you were to open your kitchen cabinets right now, about how much of the food on your shelves is over a month old? Very little? A lot? Think about this for a moment, why would food stay fresh so long out of the refrigerator? I can give you one reason: it's been heavily processed to extend the shelf life. But what does that mean nutritionally? It means your food has been sitting a long time since being picked, plucked or mixed. If we imagine our food as energy, as it's intended to be, then it's easy for us to understand that the energy our food provides starts to diminish the moment it's picked from the ground. The longer the time between packing and consumption, the less energy and nutrients we absorb from the actual food. Here's another question. If the grain in your package of crackers was harvested months before the crackers were placed on the store shelf, how much of that food's energy is left for you? Probably very little, if any. I challenge you to think of your food as energy from now on. So, the fresher it is, the more energy you get. It's a great way to determine if what we are eating is real food.

There is a famous quote by food journalist Michael Pollan that I enjoy. He says "If it came from a plant, eat it. If it was made in a plant, don't." It's such a simple rule to follow, and if you choose to live by this rule, you can be sure that your diet will be healthy. And if you want to be even more of a healthy eater, then be sure to buy your vegetables certified organic or from a local trusted farm. We live in a world with harmful toxins all around us, and food is the one source where we have some control. I will talk more about organic food a little later.

Grandma's Kitchen

Growing up, our kitchen belonged to my grandma. I would watch her spend most of the day there, chopping, slicing and preparing our family meals. Thanks to her, I learned what it meant to enjoy a wholesome, home cooked meal. So when I learned a little secret in nutrition school, it came full circle. I realized that it's actually very easy to eat healthier, just eat like my grandparents and great grandparents did. I'm serious! It's that simple. Did your forefathers eat processed food? Uh, no. They wouldn't even recognize it. So where did your great grandmother get her chocolate chip cookies? I can guarantee you it wasn't from Mrs. Fields. Here's a hint, she made them from scratch. Our great grandparents didn't shop at chain grocery stores with thousands of items lining the shelves. They grew their own vegetables and raised their own livestock. That's where their food came from. In fact, if you could travel back in time and bring your great granny here, she wouldn't recognize 90% of what is sold in the grocery store today!

We have so much to learn from our older generation. Not only about life, but about living. We've forgotten how to grow and eat real food. We have lost the traditions of healing naturally and we no longer know how to prepare a delicious meal from scratch. I just love talking to older people. Have you ever sat down with someone over the age of seventy to talk about food? I suggest you try it. Give them the opportunity to tell you what it was like to eat as a child. Ask them what their favorite food was growing up. You'll learn a lot. I remember once, a woman in her 80s approached me to ask about what kind of food she should be eating for her health. She knew I was a health coach and confessed to struggling with an out of control sweet tooth and wanted to lose weight. She asked me what kind of food is best for weight loss.

I did something she didn't expect. I asked her what kind of food she ate growing up. She look at me puzzled and then began to tell me of the freshly picked vegetables from her family garden in Germany, and how they tasted so differently from the ones she buys at the store today. Her face glowed as she reminisced about the delicious food that her mother would prepare in their family kitchen and the enjoyment they shared at the dinner table. Then I told her to simply eat that way again. To stop buying packaged food at the store and instead feast on freshly picked fruits and vegetables. Her puzzled face turned to a big smile. I could see the excitement in her eyes as she told me about the garden she wanted to plant. We chatted about organic food and natural remedies that her grandmother would use and I actually learned a lot myself.

I have had so many people ask me what a healthy diet is supposed to look like. I tell them all the same thing. You don't need to be paleo, raw, vegetarian or no carb, because everyone has different nutritional needs. But what we all need to do is go back to the basics. Fill half your plate with fresh vegetables, a serving of clean protein like organic chicken or wild salmon and a healthy fat. Enjoy more time in the kitchen, learning the art of cooking and sitting down for family meals together. Leave the laptop, iPad, or cell phone in the other room and enjoy real conversation. It's time to learn from our ancestors and eat fresh food again. We need to stop making food a quick fix for our stressful lives, but rather slow down and savor each bite. A long time ago, people were healthier. They ate real food, walked everywhere, enjoyed talking instead of watching screens, and lived a heck of a long time. They also didn't store their food in plastic, use a microwave, cook with Teflon coated pans or use plastic utensils.

Could you go back to living clean and green? I try every day, because I believe that less toxins in our food means less toxins in the body and less chance for disease. If you don't believe me, just ask my 95 year old grandmother!

80/20 Rule

I have another secret strategy called the 80/20 rule. You may have heard this term used before, but to me, it means one thing. It means that I am eating healthy foods 80 percent of the time, while the other 20 percent I allow myself to eat what would probably not be the best choice. It works great! I no longer feel deprived when I'm dining out or at a social function. I allow myself to taste whatever my desire may be. If I'm at a party and my favorite chips and dip are on the table, I take one or two bites and feel no guilt whatsoever. It works because I know that I don't eat like this all the time, and tomorrow will be different.

Am I telling you to go ahead and eat chips, fatty dips and sugar laden desserts? Absolutely not. I would prefer you didn't eat those foods at all. But there is also another aspect that goes along with eating socially. Sometimes out of courtesy, we have to eat what's served to be polite. And it's actually healthier to socialize at a party with bad foods than to stay home alone and not go at all. If you're disciplined enough to pass up all those bad foods and not feel any sort of guilt, high five to you, but don't feel bad if you're not. The truth is most of us can't resist our favorite "bad" foods when they are sitting right in front of us. And that is why the 80/20 rule works so well. You don't have to feel guilty for a little taste here and there. Because if you deprive yourself of all your favorite indulgences, you will only be left feeling unhappy, unfulfilled and wanting to binge.

However, there are a few guidelines to my 80/20 rule. If you follow them, it's simple to stay on track. As a rule of thumb, you must have at least two healthy meals on the day you eat "bad" food. That way, even though you are eating unhealthy food, your body is still getting nutrients and you won't end up feeling like crap. (Or at least as bad as you would if you ate bad all day long) The day after your cheat, make sure you start the day with a green juice, smoothie or protein shake. If you follow this rule, you won't feel sluggish or tired or gain weight. Remember, 80/20 doesn't mean you eat "bad" food *every day*; it means once in a while. Sound like an easy plan? It really is. If you want to feel even healthier, you can also try following the 90/10 rule. Yes, 90% of the time it's healthy whole foods, 10% cheats. You may need more discipline and time spent in the kitchen, but it's so worth it and you'll feel incredible!

Emotional Eating

Sometimes my 80/20 rule isn't ideal for everyone. It isn't what I recommend when working with people who are struggling with emotional eating disorders. This type of person is missing more than food to satisfy their cravings. Sometimes we crave "bad" food because we are sad, lonely, angry, or depressed. My 80/20 rule isn't a free pass to indulge yourself out of misery. It's a strategy to make eating healthy a lasting lifestyle change. If you find yourself craving bad foods regularly, then it's time to ask yourself what it is you really want. What is missing from your life? When we crave foods to make us feel better, it's time to dig deep.

Cravings happen for many reasons, stress being one of them. In order to get to the underlying cause, you must first look at your life. Ask yourself what is causing you to eat when you aren't hungry. Is it emotional pain? What thoughts are triggering your cravings? Do you feel unloved? Ashamed? Once you can identify the areas in your life where you are feeling unfulfilled, you can begin to heal and eliminate cravings. If this sounds like you, perhaps it's time to talk to an emotional eating specialist, certified health coach, or your healthcare practitioner. You don't have to suffer in silence.

Top 10 Reasons for Cravings

1. *You are dehydrated.*
2. *You are bored*
3. *You are lonely*
4. *You feel bad about your weight*
5. *Your relationship isn't fulfilling*
6. *You are stressed*
7. *You are worried*
8. *You feel overwhelmed*
9. *You feel out of control*
10. *You are depressed*

You Need Protein

If there is one food I don't want you to skip, it is protein. You need protein for building muscles, tissues, and for cell development. It's a macronutrient, meaning it provides the body with vital nutrients necessary for optimal function and health. Proteins are molecules made up of amino acids stuck together by peptide bonds. Unlike fats and sugars, we have no way to store amino acids so it's very important we eat adequate protein every day. Eating protein at every meal is also a great way to lose weight and balance blood sugar. I advise my clients with blood sugar issues to make sure to incorporate healthy fats and protein with their breakfast to keep blood sugar under control. Although you can only get complete protein through eating animal foods, it doesn't mean you *have* to eat animals. There are plenty of non-animal sources of protein to combine such as nuts, seeds, soy, green leafy vegetables, protein powders, grains, and beans. Quinoa is my favorite gluten free grain which happens to be the only whole grain to provide a complete protein.

Unfortunately, the majority of Americans today consume way too much animal protein. All that saturated fat does have negative health consequences. Plus, the meat typically comes from commercially raised animals which are fed growth hormones, antibiotics and GMO feed. Not good for your health at all. I personally stopped eating red meat, pork and lamb nearly twenty five years ago. For me, it was based on ethical as well as health related reasons. I tried being a vegetarian for a couple of years, only to become weak and anemic. I learned that my body does not absorb iron easily from non-animal sources. So my diet now includes poultry, eggs and seafood. If you decide to include animal protein in your diet, just make sure it comes from humanely raised animals, either organic, pastured or grass fed. The same goes for animal products such as eggs, cheese, butter and yogurt. I suggest you serve meat as a condiment, rather than the main course.

Got Milk?

Did you know that humans are the only mammal to continue drinking milk beyond the age of weaning. And, we are the only mammal that consumes the milk of a species other than its own. Odd, don't you think?

Just say No to GMO

Perhaps you have heard about GMOs. More and more people are learning about what they are and how they harm our health. GMOs are genetically modified organisms. They are foods that have been created in a laboratory, using science to develop a new species of plant. Sound unnatural to you? It is. How can it be healthy for humans to consume foods which are not naturally a part of our diets? It doesn't take a rocket scientist to figure that one out!

Despite my personal opinion about unnatural foods, there are scientific facts about why GMOs are dangerous. According to data from the Institute for Responsible Technology (IRT), studies on lab rats fed a diet of GMO potatoes developed potentially precancerous cell growth in the digestive tract, inhibited development of their brains, livers and testicles, partial atrophy of the liver, enlarged pancreases and intestines and had immune system damage. In another study, rats were fed Monsanto's Mon 863 Bt corn for 90 days. They showed significant changes in their blood cells, livers and kidneys, which might indicate disease. When experts demanded follow up, Monsanto used unscientific, contradictory arguments to dismiss concerns.

If you're wondering what that means for humans, there have been reported cases of farm workers and people living in areas near Bt corn fields developing skin, respiratory, and intestinal reactions while the corn is shedding pollen. This happened without eating the actual food. The bottom line is, avoid GMO foods at all cost. We know it isn't natural and has the potential for serious harm to our bodies. Currently, it's not required to label GMO food in the U.S. and Canada, so you have to be proactive. There are valid reasons that restrictions and outright bans in other countries exist. Until we can catch up with the rest of the world, the only way to protect yourself is to avoid the most common GMO food on the market today.

The Top GMO Foods to Avoid (or buy organic):

- **Corn.** About 85 percent of corn is genetically modified. And you can't just avoid corn itself, you need to read labels. Corn is a common ingredient in many processed foods, even Whole Food's brand of Corn Flakes!

- **Soy.** The most heavily genetically modified food in this country. Again, you're not safe to just avoid soy itself, but all the other processed soy products, including milk. This is especially true if you are a vegan or vegetarian and rely on soy for your protein.

- **Beet Sugar**. GMO sugar beets make up 50% of the refined sugar on the market today. You'll typically find it added as a sweetener in processed snack food and desserts. How do you avoid it? Check your labels and stay away from processed snacks.

- **Canola Oil**. Once thought of as a healthy oil to lower your cholesterol, we know differently now. Not only is it highly refined, but close to 90% of canola oil produced in the U.S. is genetically modified.

- **Milk**. Cows are often given rBGH (recombinant bovine growth hormone) to stimulate milk production. Drinking milk with rBGH has been linked to possible cancer growth leading to it being banned in the European Union, as well as in Japan, Canada, New Zealand and Australia. My advice is if you want to drink milk, only buy organic.

Organic food

Consider this, not only is the food we eat in today's world heavily processed, but the fruits and vegetables grown conventionally are sprayed with toxic chemicals. We eat these toxins. Much of the produce that you buy in the store has been bathed in pesticides. These are the same poisons that are used to kill the bugs in your garden, only a lot more potent. We should be concerned–very concerned–because our bodies are not designed to metabolize these harmful toxins. They store in our fat cells and make us sick. They can be trapped in our bodies for years, until we actively flush them out through detoxification. Because toxins tend to accumulate in the fat cells, studies have shown that these toxins in our bodies can also contribute to weight gain.

Many years ago I worked at the National Headquarters of the Sierra Club. It was an eye opening experience. Even back in the late 1980s, the Sierra Club was actively fighting to stop pesticides from polluting the planet. It was the first time I realized that harmful chemicals were being sprayed on the fruits and vegetables that we ate. I learned that strawberries and apples had the highest concentration of pesticides, and to boycott grapes because of the unfair migrant worker conditions. It's hard to imagine that was 25 years ago. Here we are today, still fighting the same battles. Still dealing with pesticides and unfair labor practices. Only now we have more crops being sprayed and a new bad guy...GMOs.

I would love to tell you to buy only organic produce, but I know it's not realistic. Most of us live on a tight budget. Yes, organic food does cost a bit more, but isn't your health worth it? If you're on a limited budget, you can still protect your health by buying "the dirtiest" fruits and vegetables in the organic section. The foods listed on the "Dirty Dozen" are the most heavily sprayed with pesticides, and ones you should always buy organic. This is especially important if you serve them to your children or eat them often.

Fast Food Fact

The junk food industry spends millions of dollars to develop the perfect combination of sugar, fat, and salt to appeal to your taste buds. That's why you crave certain bad food. They have it down to a science.

Dirty Dozen Plus ™

Apples
Strawberries
Grapes
Celery
Peaches
Spinach
Sweet Bell Peppers
Nectarines (imported)
Cucumber
Cherry Tomatoes
Snap Peas (imported)
Potatoes
Hot Peppers
Kale and Collard Greens

If you want to learn more about ways to reduce toxins in your life, I recommend visiting the Environmental Working Group website, www.ewg.org. You can also find out which foods are on the **Clean 15**™ list.

Chapter 7
Good Fat is Your Friend

If you are one of the millions of people who are afraid to eat an avocado, eggs or real butter, for fear that it will raise your bad cholesterol and put you at risk for heart disease, then this is your day to rejoice! I'm here to tell you that it is simply not true. Yes, there are bad fats out there. But there are also healthy, good for you, necessary fats too. And it's time to stop being afraid of fat and realize that fat can be your best friend.

Beginning in the late 1970s, the U.S. government issued a recommendation for Americans to eat a low fat diet for heart health. Based on no real studies, the dietary guidelines warned us that all saturated fat would lead to heart disease. It was believed that high cholesterol was the leading cause of heart attacks and strokes. Thankfully, we know differently now, and fat is back on the table! Unfortunately, thanks to all the low fat and fat free foods that saturated the market back then, we as a nation, started to get fatter. Only today are we beginning to connect the dots. While people were avoiding eating anything with fat, they were also filling their bellies with loads of refined white carbohydrates, like fat free cookies, cinnamon raisin bagels, blueberry muffins and a lot of wheat bread. We became a nation of carbohydrate addicts. And I was one of them! I remember eating my granola cereal or dry onion bagel for breakfast, skipping the butter. I would pass up avocado on my salad and eat bread sticks instead. Or indulge in a big plate of pasta with tomato sauce for dinner and stayed away from any type of fat and fattening oils. I used to wonder why I needed to exercise so much, just to keep my weight down. Well, now I know. All those fat free refined carbohydrates like bread, crackers and pasta, simply turned into sugar the minute it entered my bloodstream. Which triggered my pancreas to release more insulin and get ready to store fat.

Thank goodness the 80s are over. The fashion can keep trying to come back, but please, not the food! It's taken three decades but we finally figured out that we need fat in our diet. Not only do our bodies crave it, but it's essential for our brain to work efficiently. You may not know this, but our brains are made up of 60% fat. That's a lot of fat! Perhaps it also explains why the 80s wasn't known as the most intellectual generation. (Just kidding) But before you run out and celebrate with a meal of sausage and eggs, there are some things you need to know about fat.

First, you only want to eat healthy fats. It's important to learn the difference between healthy fat and bad fat, because unhealthy fats will clog your arteries and contribute to increased "bad" cholesterol. The type of good fats I'm talking about are monounsaturated and polyunsaturated, plus a few saturated fats, in moderation. These are the fats found in nuts, seeds, avocados, and cold water fish. They are rich in Omega 3 fatty acids and help lower inflammation in the body.

On the other hand, the number one fat you do NOT want to eat are known as trans fats. This is the kind of fat you find in processed frozen foods like pizza or pies; it's in margarine, packaged snacks, at fast food restaurants, and store bought baked goods. Trans fats are very unhealthy oils high in inflammatory causing Omega 6 fatty acids. Trans fats are made by mixing hydrogen with vegetable oils so they can stay solid even at room temperature. Word of caution, you must be careful of product labels that claim "no trans fats" because according to the FDA, manufacturers do not have to list trans fats on the label if the amount used is less than 1%. And any percent is still too much. Why it's very important to always read labels!

Here's an easy way to tell if a product has trans fats. If the label lists any hydrogenated oils (even partially) then don't buy it. Those are trans fats. If you're wondering what is so bad about trans fats, they contribute to heart disease, cause dangerous plaque to build up in your arteries and increase your risk for type 2 diabetes. They also clog your liver and cause inflammatory disease. If the FDA recognizes that trans fats need to be banned, you can be sure it's *very* bad for you.

Maybe you're not quite ready to start eating only real, fresh food. Then be sure to make a habit of reading product labels. The fewer ingredients listed on the label, the better. The worst two ingredients to avoid are partially hydrogenated oils and high fructose corn syrup. If the item you are looking at has it on the label, put it back!

Good fats and oils

- Cold water fish (wild caught salmon, sardines, and anchovies)
- Avocado
- Cold Pressed Extra Virgin Olive Oil
- Extra Virgin Coconut oil
- Sesame oil
- Avocado oil
- Flax seeds and oil
- Organic butter (from grass fed cows)
- Ghee (clarified butter)
- Nuts (walnuts, cashews, pecans, almonds, macadamia, brazil nuts)
- Almond butter, cashew butter and sunflower butter (unsweetened)
- Raw seeds (pumpkin, sunflower, sesame)
- Chia seeds
- Hemp seeds
- Shredded coconut (unsweetened)

Chapter 8
Sugar, the Real Enemy

Okay, here is another big secret. If you stop eating sugar and refined carbohydrates you *will* start to lose weight...and the unhealthy kind of fat that stores around your waist. You may know it as the dreaded belly fat. This is the type of fat which is linked to heart attacks, atherosclerosis, and heart disease. Why? Because the fat is stored around your waist and closer to your heart. Makes sense, doesn't it? Another reason why it's so important to lose excess belly fat. And, eliminating sugar and refined carbohydrates is the quickest way to see a difference.

Please listen carefully, sugar is your enemy! We now know that sugar is responsible for not only causing obesity, but also high blood pressure, dementia, type 2 diabetes, vascular disease, colorectal cancer and even osteoporosis. I know, giving up sugar is no easy task. Especially for us stressed out and busy women! We have come to rely on sugar for energy and most likely are addicted to the oh-so-lovely sugar high. So yes, it will take commitment and hard work to kick the sugar habit. But whether you are struggling with your weight or not, you will be amazed at how great your body and mind will feel once you stop feeding it with sugar. It may sound contradictory to everything you've learned about sugar—that we need it to give us energy—but we get plenty of energy from the natural sugar found in fruits and vegetables. Sugary snacks may leave you feeling energetic at first, but it's only temporary, and the surge is followed by a big crash. You are then left feeling even more tired than before you ate the sugary snack.

Perhaps you are confused about what are the healthiest natural sweeteners. You're not alone. Many wellness experts disagree about which ones are good or bad. And so are the nutritionists. It seems everyone has a different opinion on which are the healthiest sweeteners. I've listed my personal favorites based on everything I have learned over the years. But let me add that I encourage you to use as little added sweetener as possible. And please, avoid anything with high fructose corn syrup! More harmful than white refined sugar, HFCS is derived from GMO corn and contributes directly to type 2 diabetes. Of course, too much of any sugar is never a good thing and eventually can lead to obesity and heart disease. It stresses your body and causes an imbalance in your blood sugar, and also causes you to age faster. Through the process of glycation, your cells age faster and so does your skin. If you need another reason to give up sugar, consider the damage it's doing to your youthful appearance!

However, when it comes to natural sugar versus artificial sweeteners, it's pretty clear to me. Stay as far away from artificial sweeteners as you can! You won't hear it talked about in the news, but not only are artificial sweeteners unsafe, they actually make you gain more weight over time. Marketed as a low calorie, sugar free alternative, artificial sweeteners are up to 200 times sweeter than table sugar. That excessive sweetness tricks your brain into wanting more sugar, so you end up consuming more sweet foods. Which means more calories are consumed leading to weight gain. In fact, one study concluded that people who consumed artificial sweeteners had a higher BMI (body mass index) than those who didn't.

If you are living with elevated blood sugar (pre diabetes) or have been diagnosed with type 2 diabetes, you may be wondering how do I still enjoy dessert? I suggest you stay away from artificial sweeteners. If you really must have sweets, try sweet vegetables or low sugar fruit. A low glycemic alternative is liquid stevia or if you don't like the aftertaste, try a teaspoon of pure maple syrup or molasses. Both are delicious sweeteners and won't spike your blood sugar. I like raw honey and maple syrup because they taste delicious and offer the most nutrients. An equally important food group to avoid, aside from table sugar, is refined white carbohydrates like bread, rice, pasta, cookies and crackers. These foods will metabolize to sugar as soon as they enter your bloodstream. In fact, according to William Davis, MD, the author of "Wheat Belly," when you eat two slices of wheat bread, it raises your blood sugar as if you ate a candy bar. Imagine that! Unless you are an athlete and about to run a marathon, you just don't need all those carbohydrates.

I know, you're wondering if it is really possible to give up sugar. I believe you can. At least to the point that you will feel a difference and not feel deprived. How do I know this? I've seen it happen with my clients and also with myself. If you don't think you need to give up sugar, consider this, it's robbing you of your energy, causing you to age faster, making you fat, and raising your risk for heart disease and type 2 diabetes. The American Heart Association suggests Americans consume as little as possible and set a limit of no more than 24 grams per day for women and 36 grams per day for men. An easy way to gauge your sugar consumption is to remember there are 4 grams of sugar in one teaspoon.

My Favorite Natural Sweeteners

- ♥ Stevia, raw or liquid
- ♥ Raw honey
- ♥ Molasses
- ♥ Pure maple syrup
- ♥ Dried dates or date sugar
- ♥ Coconut palm sugar

The Fake Stuff

I'm going to say it again: please stay away from artificial sweeteners. They may sound like a great low calorie alternative to sugar, but know that they are manufactured from chemicals that may actually raise your risk of diabetes. Sold on the market as the perfect alternative to sugar, they are far from being good for you. If you think the FDA allowed aspartame (NutraSweet and Equal) on the market in 1983 because it's safe to consume, think again. It took nine years and several rejections by the FDA for the manufacturer to finally get approval to distribute it on the market. And still, many studies have shown a link to cancer and other health related side effects. Here's my big problem with artificial sweeteners. They are made from chemicals. In fact, the first artificial sweetener was discovered in a laboratory by accident. Chemist James M. Schlatter who worked for G.D. Searle, was developing a drug to treat peptic ulcer disease when he spilled one of the chemicals called aspartame onto his finger. While licking it off (yes he did), he realized it had a sweet taste. And there you have it, Equal was born.

Let me also point out that artificial sweeteners are up to 200 times sweeter than real sugar. When you consume artificial sweeteners, your taste buds are flooded with excessive sweetness and your pancreas releases glucose into your blood stream, ready to unlock the cells and let the sugar in. But wait... when no sugar shows up the body is confused and the excess glucose is stored as fat. I bet you never knew this little side effect. Over time, your body begins craving more sugar in desperation for energy. If that's not enough to change your mind, newer studies are now showing that ingesting artificial sweeteners will start to change the health of your gut flora. A healthy gut is made up of both good bacteria and bad, which need to be in perfect balance, but when we consume chemicals such as artificial sweeteners, it seems to kill off the good bacteria. Eventually, you are lowering your metabolism and causing the body to hold onto fat.

Eat Less Sugar, You are Already Sweet Enough!

So, have I convinced you to give up sugar? How about for just a week? Think you can do it? Believe it or not, you will start to have more energy once you kick your sugar habit. One of the first changes I noticed after giving up my Starbucks Vanilla Latte daily habit was that I started to have more energy in the afternoon. Also, my taste buds started to change. It seemed the less sugar I ate, the sweeter my food became. Sounds bizarre, doesn't it? But it's true. I can now taste the sweetness in nuts, root vegetables, and even 90% dark chocolate. My taste buds have actually come alive with the absence of added sugar.

The best way to give up sugar is to just go cold turkey. It takes about 21 days for your body to lose the sweet cravings. Eventually your taste buds will change and what used to be your favorite sugary treats will taste too sweet for you to tolerate. Believe me, I've seen it happen to every one of my clients after they curbed their sugar consumption. And the great news is that you will develop a new appreciation for sweet fruits and vegetables. Your palate will improve and you'll find store bought candy bars to taste artificial. By giving up sugar for just one week, you will begin to taste the sweetness of an almond and be surprised at how yummy a sweet potato with cinnamon can be!

I understand if you absolutely cannot give up sugar cold turkey. After all, sugar was once considered a drug! In fact, one study of lab mice who were given the choice or either sugar or cocaine, chose the sugar every time. That's a powerful message. Sure, we aren't mice, but our brain chemistry pretty much works the same way. Maybe now you won't be so hard on yourself if your brain doesn't want to give up the sweet feeling you get when you eat sugar.

But before you throw your hands up in the air and say "I give up" here are some strategies you can try to slowly quit sugar. I suggest first gradually reducing the amount of added sugar you consume every day. Start to replace it with some of the healthier natural sweeteners on my list. Begin to eat more sour foods, like lemons and limes. Drink a glass of water with lemon juice every morning before eating breakfast. Make sure you are including protein rich food into your diet and eating adequate fiber to keep you feeling full. By following these tips, you'll have less sugar cravings. But remember, I never want you to use artificial sweeteners. They are absolutely forbidden!

Sugar is eight times more addictive than cocaine.

Dr. Mark Hyman, author of "The Blood Sugar Solution"

Watch Out for Hidden Sugar!

Guess what, sugar is added to many processed foods. So it's always smart to read ingredient labels. Here are some foods you wouldn't suspect are laden with sugar.

- Salad dressings (especially fat free)
- Flavored yogurts (including Greek Style)
- Ketchup
- Spaghetti sauce
- Fruit juice
- Low fat food
- Gluten free baked goods
- Vitamin water (31 grams per serving!)
- Store bought "healthy" fruit smoothies

Remember, there are 4 grams of sugar in one teaspoon. You may be surprised to learn that your favorite healthy juice has five or more teaspoons of sugar per serving. That's a heck of a lot of sugar!

Wheat and Gluten

I'm not going to go in depth about the side effects of eating wheat and gluten. There are plenty of books on the subject if you want to learn more. But I do want to mention it because it's a popular topic right now. For those who don't know, gluten is a protein found in grains such as wheat, barley, rye, couscous and kamut. It's the "glue" that holds flour together to make breads, cookies and other baked goods. As we learn more, many people are discovering sensitivities or intolerances to gluten, most likely because the wheat we eat today is not the wheat of our ancestors. There is some speculation that this modern day hybridized wheat is not well tolerated by our bodies. Gluten has even been linked to brain health and cognitive function, as discussed in the book "Grain Brain" by David Perlmutter, MD. If you want to learn more about gluten, there is also a wealth of information available online at www.theglutensummit.com. You will be surprised to learn how many symptoms and ailments are linked to gluten intolerances and sensitivities.

Functional medicine and nutrition experts have even linked gluten to the development of a leaky gut, also known as intestinal permeability–a condition that happens when the lining of the gut is irritated by an inflammatory response, causing small holes or tears to form in the digestive tract. As food particles, debris and toxins pass through the intestines, some may leak through the holes and enter the bloodstream. This triggers an autoimmune response, which can lead to gastrointestinal problems such as abdominal bloating, excessive gas and cramps, fatigue, food sensitivities, joint pain, skin rashes, and autoimmunity.

If you're wondering why wheat and gluten ended up in the chapter on sugar, it's because processed carbohydrates are a leading cause of obesity in this country. You see, a slice of wheat bread will raise your blood sugar in the same way as a candy bar. Yes, you heard me right. Processed carbohydrates like bread, pasta, crackers, and noodles are basically sugar inside your body.

These starchy carbohydrates are more harmful to you than eating bacon and butter. Remember, fat is not your enemy, sugar is! I personally found that my weight stabilized and the muffin top disappeared when I gave up eating breads and pasta. It was the one big change that has made a difference in my energy too.

I still eat grains and carbohydrates on occasion, but I feel a significant difference in my body when I do. I first noticed this after bingeing on sourdough bread, homemade pie, and too many cookies over the holidays. Within days my joints were swollen and painful, my energy was low and my head was in a brain fog. It was a very noticeable difference in my health. Up until that point, I knew that gluten was not good, but had no idea how bad it was *for me*. After experiencing my body's inflammatory response, I decided to give it up 95% of the time. I suggest you try eliminating wheat and gluten for a few weeks. Then reintroduce it for a couple of days and see how you feel. You may be surprised.

Gluten Free Grains

- Amaranth
- Buckwheat
- Corn (non GMO)
- Millet
- Quinoa
- Rice (brown or black)
- Teff

Chapter 9
A Healthy Gut

It's an exciting time in nutrition and wellness right now. We are learning more and more about the function of the human body than ever before. Especially our amazing digestive system. In the years ahead, be on the lookout for clinical studies on the health of our gut and it's relation to the balance of bacteria. We are learning every day the importance of good bacteria in the gut, and how more than digestive disease is affected by an imbalance of this vital organ. Researchers are discovering that an imbalance in our gut can result in many more symptoms other than an upset stomach or constipation. The balance of our intestinal flora determines the health of our brains, immune function, and metabolic rate. It's simply amazing.

It's hard to imagine that every one of us has trillions of microorganisms living in our body at any moment. We need them to survive. Our good and bad bacteria must be in perfect balance in order to keep us healthy and feeling good. The gut is their primary home, and when we eat poorly, take antibiotics, and live in stress, we are not only killing off our good bacteria, we are changing the delicate balance of the gut. We end up having more bad bacteria, and that's when symptoms can arise such as IBS, chronic diarrhea, constipation, belly bloat, or foggy brain. Recent studies are now suggesting that there is a gut-brain connection. Ever hear the saying "listen to your gut?" Well, it's not as far-fetched as you may have thought. Our gut health is now being linked to mental health, mood, and cognitive function. Research is exploring the connection of the gut microbiome with autism, anxiety, depression and immune health. With so much new information coming out about the health of the gut, it makes sense to pay attention and start feeding it the right foods!

Why You Need Probiotics

One very easy way to maintain gut health is to take a daily probiotic supplement. Replacing your good bacteria on a regular basis will help heal your gut and encourage the good bacteria to colonize and stick around, crowding out the bad bacteria and keeping your intestinal flora in balance. Why is this so important? Remember, our bodies are made up of trillions of bacteria. In fact, these living organisms make up most of who we are. Yes, we are walking bacteria! Because we live in a world with chronic stress, eat a heavily acidic diet and take too many antibiotics, we need to be replacing the good bacteria being destroyed every day. I predict that probiotics are soon to be as common as taking a daily multivitamin. We need them for proper digestion and to keep our immune system working efficiently.

Choosing a probiotic supplement can be confusing, with so many new products hitting the market all the time. When buying a probiotic, it's best to find one sold in the refrigerated section, since live cultures are sensitive to heat and can die. Ideally, you want several strains of bacteria, including both Lactobacillus and Bifidobacterium, and have at least 10 to 20 billion CFUs (live bacteria) per serving.

Fermented Vegetables

Another great way to balance your gut and restore healthy bacteria is by incorporating fermented foods into your diet. These foods have lots of wonderful healthy bacteria and are very bioavailable. Fermented foods, also called cultured foods, have been around for thousands of years. Many cultures have long known about their health-promoting benefits. Cultured foods are vegetables which have been fermented in their brine and given time to form healthy bacteria. They are a great way to maintain a healthy gut flora and should be a part of everyone's diet. My favorite fermented foods are Kim Chee, a spicy Korean dish made from fermented cabbage, and the classic Sauerkraut, but make sure it's raw and refrigerated. If you are the type of person who loves to experiment in the kitchen, go ahead and prepare your own fermented vegetables at home. It's easy and fun!

Food Combining for Optimal Digestion

PROTEINS

(poultry, fish, meat, dairy, soybean, eggs, nuts, seeds, coconut)

OR

CARBOHYDRATES

(beans, grains, lentils, potatoes, pumpkin, squash)

WITH

NON STARCHY VEGETABLES

(asparagus, broccoli, lettuces, kale, Cabbage, cucumber, collards, eggplant, green beans, leeks, onions, spinach, sprouts, sweet peppers, tomatoes, turnips, zucchini)

FATS AND OILS

(avocado, butter, lard, nut oils, olive oil, sesame oil)

Fruit is best eaten alone on an empty stomach

Chapter 10
Detox the Junk

Even with the healthiest diet and cleanest lifestyle, we all accumulate toxic junk in our bodies. Unless you live in a bubble, the simple act of walking outside and breathing the air exposes you to toxins. That's why it's important to clean out the pipes and detoxify your body on a regular basis. The truth is, we live in a modern world, which means we are surrounded by technology, machinery, chemicals and pesticides. All of those chemicals have the potential to build up in our bodies. We eat food that has been sprayed with pesticides, drink water with heavy metals and contaminants, live in houses decorated with furniture treated with fire retardants, and put personal products on our bodies which have hundreds of chemicals in them. Yes, we live in a toxic world.

So what do we do? We certainly can't live in a bubble. It's not practical…or fun! Well, we nourish our bodies with the healthiest foods possible, eliminate as many toxins as we can from our life, and detox our bodies on a regular basis. Consider this, every food you consume, every breath you take, and everything you touch during your day brings with it contaminants. This constant barrage forces your liver to work hard detoxifying your body. Because there is no way to avoid all of these toxins as they build up, our bodies have to work harder and harder to process them. If we never stop and give the body a rest our liver becomes congested and we feel unbalanced. When your body is out of balance you can experience fatigue, indigestion, hormonal issues, depression, poor concentration, and sluggish bowels. When your body is balanced, you will experience more energy, clarity, a general feeling of vitality and lightness, regular bowel movements and no more brain fog.

I'm a strong believer in seasonal detox programs. It's important to give the digestion a rest and allow it to naturally cleanse and reset. In my health coaching practice, I lead two seasonal group cleanses; one in the spring, and one in the fall. These are the ideal times of the year to support the body's own natural detoxification process. By doing a detox, you are helping the body move toxins through the lymphatic system (our drain pipes) and eventually out of your body. You give your body a rest, and you also support proper digestion which is the key to permanent weight loss and a healthy immune function. If you've ever tried hard to lose weight and failed, it could very well be a sign of toxic overload. Remember, your body truly does crave a perfect balance.

Top Food Allergens

These are the foods most likely to cause an inflammatory reaction. It's important to avoid these foods while on a cleanse or detox program.

- Wheat/gluten
- Dairy
- Corn
- Eggs
- Beef
- Pork
- Shellfish
- Soy
- Peanuts
- Refined Sugars
- Alcohol

Food Preparation Made Simple

Okay, so you are ready to eat clean! I know what it's like to be a busy woman with no time to cook. It's quite a challenge. Not having time is the most common reason we give up eating clean or attempting to prepare wholesome food. Over the years, I've learned how to simplify my cooking and take short cuts in preparation time. I rarely make big elaborate meals, yet my food is still tasty, healthy and simple to prepare. There is no reason you need to feel anxious about making a nice meal.

If you are the type of person who struggles in the kitchen, don't panic! By following my simple strategies, you will get better at pulling together quick and easy meals in no time. Like anything else, it takes practice, but you may surprise yourself and not only become skilled but start to really enjoy preparing nourishing, tasty meals.

Here are my strategies for the busy woman in the kitchen.

♥ Keep it simple! Don't get overwhelmed by feeling you have to make a gourmet meal. A simple stir fry is my favorite quick meal. Just heat a tablespoon of coconut oil (or avocado oil) in a skillet and add some minced garlic and ginger until softened (watch carefully so that the garlic doesn't burn), then add your preferred chopped vegetables. Once the veggies, garlic, and ginger are soft and stirred together, remove them to a plate to keep warm. Then add a protein of your choice to your pan and a little more oil if you need it. Protein generally cooks in about 6 to 8 minutes. Try not to overcook it but always follow the proper temperature guidelines for meat and poultry. Add your veggies back in to warm and voila: you have a fabulous, healthy meal!

♥ Find recipes that have five ingredients or less. Simple meals mean less bloating and more nourishment. This will also keep you eating healthier, since you'll be using mostly fresh ingredients.

♥ If you are always on the go, you can prep your meals on weekends. You can also make soups ahead and freeze or make a large batch of vegetables, protein and brown rice for the week.

♥ A big time saver is to buy pre-chopped, pre-sliced, and pre-shredded produce. You can easily find pre-packaged shredded carrots, cabbage, brussel sprouts, broccoli slaw, chopped onions, sliced mushrooms and pre-washed spinach and kale in most stores today.

♥ Shop and do all your prep on the weekends. If you want to save time during the week, do the shopping on a weekend and as soon as you come home, spend an hour to wash, chop, and place your vegetables in containers before putting them away.

♥ My favorite healthy meal is a large green salad with lots of colorful vegetables. Just chop a big batch of veggies and store in the fridge for assembling quick salads during the week. You can also have them ready to go in BPA-free plastic containers or glass Mason jars, with the dressing stored separately. I like to buy the organic salad greens and add my own dressing of fresh lemon juice and olive oil.

♥ **Dining Out Tips**: Choose simple dishes like steamed vegetables with chicken or fish, a large green salad with colorful veggies, some protein and a dressing made of lemon juice and olive oil, or order a bowl of homemade vegetable soup (not creamed).

Build a Simple Salad

- 2 cups organic mixed greens
- Choice of protein or 1/2 cup beans of your choice
- Chopped raw or lightly steamed vegetables (lots of color!) I like red and orange bell peppers, red onions, broccoli, artichoke hearts, carrots, asparagus)
- Simple dressing made with juice of one lemon, extra virgin olive oil, sea salt and pepper
- 2 tbsp. healthy fat, such as sliced avocado, sunflower seeds or pumpkin seeds
- Dried cranberries as a topping (optional)

Put your salad in the refrigerator (sans dressing) and it will be ready to take to work the next day or for dinner when you get home. Perfect for those days with no time to prepare a healthy meal.

Practice Mindful Eating

Slowing down and paying attention to your meal aids in digestion and prevents you from overeating. Practice these simple tips:

- ♥ Chew your food thoroughly
- ♥ Put the fork down between bites
- ♥ Savor the flavors
- ♥ Stop eating when you are 80% full

PART THREE
Love Yourself

"Love is the great miracle cure.
Loving ourselves works miracles in our lives."

— *Louise L. Hay*

Chapter 11
Putting Yourself First

I believe that taking time for oneself is *the* most important thing a woman can do to stay healthy. Unfortunately, it's typically the last thing we do as mothers, wives, partners, or daughters. Sure, going to the gym is good for your health, but how often do you take time to do something relaxing, fun, or nurturing? As natural caregivers, we often spend our days running around taking care of everyone and everything. By the end of the day, it seems we can barely find the energy to brush our teeth and wash our face. We have given so much of ourselves to everyone else, that there is nothing left for us. I'm sure you have realized by now, that if we don't take care of ourselves, how will we be able to keep taking care of others?

News flash! It's NOT selfish to put yourself first. The idea of doing something nice for yourself before everyone else may sound selfish, but believe me, it is not at all. It's important for us to take time to turn off our sympathetic nervous system and keep cortisol levels low. If you consider exercise as your primary way to unwind, that's great. But remember, you still need to practice a calming exercise that turns down the cortisol in your body and allows it to reset and relax.

In functional medicine, most practitioners will agree that disease usually has a root cause; it doesn't just appear out of nowhere. That's because our body begins to get sick many years before we ever experience any physical symptoms. By the time we feel sick and go to the doctor, most of the damage has already been done. Which is why I like to say we don't have a health care system, but rather a sick care system. Traditional western medicine is currently lacking in holistic wellness programs necessary to help prevent disease. Most patients today are simply instructed to fill a prescription and go on with life, rather than spend an hour discussing lifestyle, nutrition and mental wellness.

So, how does illness relate to putting yourself first? Taking care of you plays a key role in your health. If you don't take care of yourself, who will? For many of us moms, we would give our last bit of food to our child, we would freeze to keep our kids warm, and there is no question we would lose sleep to comfort our sick baby. There is nothing we wouldn't do or sacrifice for our children. But yet, it feels selfish for us to take time away from helping others to do something nurturing for ourselves. Have you ever felt guilty for taking a day to be alone? I certainly have!

I still can't believe that my first (real) alone time after my son was born didn't happen until his first day of preschool. Until that day, all of my time was devoted to his care. That first day being alone, with only a few hours to myself, was such an awkward feeling. It had been so long that I forgot what it felt like to have time for *me*. I didn't know what to do. I had sworn that I would not go home and clean for three hours, but you guessed it, I did just that. I went home and spent those three glorious hours to myself cleaning the darn house from top to bottom. Because I just didn't know what else to do! Sounds pretty pathetic, doesn't it. Unfortunately, I'm not the only woman guilty of doing housework when I should be doing something fun. Because that's what mothers do. Of course, over time, I learned to appreciate those few solitary hours, just a few days a week, and began to do nurturing things for myself. Just those few hours a week alone probably saved me from going insane!

We busy women like to think we are indestructible, that we can just keep going and going without consequences. Oh, how that kind of thinking will get us in trouble. Big trouble. I used to think that way too. Being an older mom with a very active child and parents who were elderly and frail, I had my share of challenges. But I felt I had nothing to fear. After all, what did I need? I had a child, my parents, a husband and house full of pets. As long as everyone else was happy and getting what they needed, I thought I was happy. But deep down, I wasn't. How could I be happy if I didn't even have time to take a relaxing soak in my tub? It became pretty clear that not taking care of myself was turning me into a not-very-happy person to be around. I was walking around feeling tired and frustrated. It certainly wasn't good for my health. But as I started to be a little more selfish, my family started to benefit as well. Instead of feeling frustrated and angry all the time, my moods were more stable and I felt happier. Of course, it's no big surprise, because when we take care of ourselves, everyone around us benefits. Ever hear the phrase, "happy wife, happy life?" Now go do something nice for yourself!

Try this simple exercise to help you find joy in each day. Bonus: You'll have to spend a few minutes by yourself.

Give Gratitude

Buy yourself a beautiful journal.

For the next two weeks, find time in the early morning or before bed to write down at least three things you are grateful for that happened that day. Then write one thing you are grateful for that has happened in your life.

By the end of the two weeks, you will see that noting the positive in your life will make you feel calmer and happier.

Chapter 12
Fall Madly in Love with You

There is nothing you can do for others that is more loving than loving yourself. Because when you love yourself, your heart is open, your compassion is bigger, you bring happiness to others and you are a more loving person. So don't ever feel guilty for loving yourself. You work hard. You are a giving person. You deserve it.

My Favorite Self Love Rituals

Epsom Salt Bath
One of my favorite ways to relax. Add ½ cup of Epsom salt, ½ cup baking soda, and a few drops of lavender essential oil to a warm bath and soak for 20 minutes. Epsom salt relaxes the body, detoxifies the liver, and provides your body with the mineral magnesium, which is necessary for optimal relaxation, digestion, detox and overall health.

Massage
Massage is a wonderful way to pamper yourself. It relaxes your body, lowers cortisol and keeps your lymphatic pathways flowing. I schedule a massage for once a month, it's my ultimate self-love ritual. Try a hot stone or aromatherapy massage for even greater relaxation.

Go for a Hike
There is nothing more peaceful than being in nature. Did you know that just looking at beautiful scenery can improve your health? When I need to unwind, I leash up my dog and head to the trails. Taking a moderate one or two hour hike is just as therapeutic as going to the spa…and it cost nothing!

Get a Pedicure
The very first self-love ritual I started. Pamper your feet and you'll be walking on air.

Buy Something Pretty
I'm not a shopper at all, but who doesn't love finding a pretty dress, pair of cute shoes, or beautiful handbag? My favorite stores to browse are consignment. It's like raiding a fashionista's closet!

Practice Yoga
Yes, I feel like yoga is a form of self-love, because yoga makes me feel like I've just been to the spa.

Take 10
Sometimes we just need to stop and do nothing. Give yourself permission to spend 10 minutes of quiet reflection time.

Get a Haircut
Book an appointment at the salon to have your hair cut, washed and conditioned followed by a scalp massage and blow dry. Later in the evening, go out for a yummy dinner and show off your expertly styled hair!

Eat Dark Chocolate
Yes, chocolate is healthy for you and tastes divine. The darker the better too. It also has properties that stimulate the brain to produce a feeling of being in love. No wonder we crave it!

Chapter 13
Beauty from the Inside Out

I don't think any woman looks forward to gray hair and wrinkles. (Well, I do have one friend) But the vast majority of us would love to maintain our youthful appearance for as long as possible. At one time in our lives, we paid too much money for a miracle face cream, which claimed that it would reverse the signs of aging and make your skin look radiant and flawless. Of course, it didn't really work. Sure, your face may have smelled like a rose garden and it felt so silky on your skin, but face it (pun intended), it wasn't a miracle cream. Your skin is still aging.

Why is it that we try so hard to find the right facial cream, yet we don't really pay attention to what we are putting inside our bodies? Have you ever stopped to wonder if there is a link between what you eat and how your skin ages? I'm not suggesting that what we put on our skin isn't important, because it is. Your skin absorbs lotions and creams, so we need to be careful of the chemicals in our products. What I mean is the food we eat also impacts the condition of our skin. Most women will buy expensive facial creams and make up, yet live on a diet of sugar, carbohydrates and alcohol. A very bad combination for your skin by the way. Throw in a stressful life and lack of sleep, and you have the perfect recipe for premature aging and poor skin.

I'm often complimented on how young I look for my age. It's always very sweet to hear, but honestly I do. At age 52, I can easily get away with telling people I'm ten years younger. Sure, I can attribute my youthful appearance to my wonderful genes, but living a healthy lifestyle for most of my life has also been a big reason. Besides looking young, I have abundant energy and a clear mind. I can honestly say that I *feel* younger today than I did in my 30s and 40s. No joke! I may not be able to abuse my body by drinking wine all night and bounce back the very next day, but my daily energy and mental focus is a hundred times greater.

And you know what: *you* can feel this way too. Despite being a busy and stressed out woman (which you will work on changing, right) you have the power to improve your life and slow down the aging process. In fact, when you start eating clean, reducing your stress, cutting back on sugar, and sleeping more, you will start to see a reversal in signs of aging. Sound good? You won't need to spend hundreds of dollars on anti-aging products anymore. Just follow my tips and make simple lifestyle changes–your skin will start glowing and you'll feel like a million bucks.

So, where do you begin? First, eat a healthy diet. Incorporate lots of clean protein, good fats, and vegetables. And be sure to kick your sugar habit! Give up processed food, which is aging your skin at light speed. Start your morning with a healthy green smoothie and drink plenty of water. Finally, check the ingredient labels on your beauty products. Get rid of anything with harmful chemicals!

Beauty Boosting Foods

Avocado
Beets
Berries; blueberries, blackberries, raspberries
Carrots
Celery
Cucumbers
Green leafy vegetables; spinach, kale, lettuces
Lemons
Sweet potatoes
Tomatoes
Wild salmon

Chapter 14
Circle of Life

When I was in nutrition school, we learned about Primary Foods ™ and secondary foods. Primary foods are the things in our lives that nourish us but are not the food we eat. They are the parts of our lives which feed our souls. Secondary foods are the foods we eat. It's the nutrition we need to sustain our life. Yet, it's crucial for both of these "foods" to be in balance, because when we are not fulfilled in one area of our lives or the other, we cannot experience perfect health. Primary food and secondary food are part of what was called "the circle of life." It's all the parts of our life which need to be balanced in order to be truly healthy.

If you were to look at your life right now, what part of you feels unfulfilled? What parts of your life make you satisfied and what parts are lacking? Your goal is to have all the parts of your life feel close to equal in satisfaction and importance. The concept of balance is taught in many ancient cultures and natural healing. Our lives should not only be about our work, our relationships, our spirituality, the food we eat or how much we exercise. If we want to have a balanced and fulfilling life, we need to be rich in all of those areas.

Using the following diagram, make a dot on each line indicating your satisfaction with that part of your life. The closer the dot is to the center, the more unfulfilled you are, the closer to the outer edge, the more satisfied you feel. After you finish placing all your dots, make a line connecting them together. What does your line look like? Do they make a nice circle, or look jagged and disconnected? Your personal circle will tell you what areas of your life need improvement.

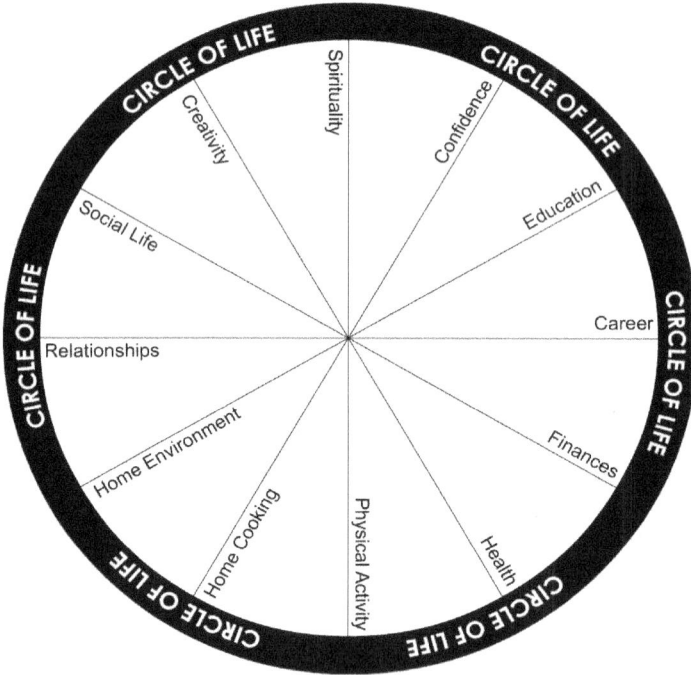

© 2011 Integrative Nutrition Inc.

My Circle

Fulfilled: _____

_____

Needs Improvement: _____

_____

PART FOUR
Glow into Your Golden Years

"Plant your own garden and decorate your own soul
instead of waiting for someone to bring you flowers."
— Veronica A. Shoffstall

Chapter 15
My Healthy Aging Tips

For most of my life, I've had a personal interest in anything related to healthy aging. I figure if I make it to old age, I want to be in the best shape possible. I don't plan to be in a wheel chair, hooked up to machines, or confined to a bed. I want to be one of those centenarians who is still thriving at age 103!

Get Sleep

Ah, I can hear you. Sleep, you say? What is that? If you're like nearly every busy woman I know, you are not sleeping enough. If I told you that getting a good night's sleep was critical for slowing down the aging process would you listen? Sleeping Beauty was on to something. Not only do we need restorative sleep for our cells and tissue to regenerate, we need it to reset our adrenals, balance our hormones, keep our metabolism working efficiently (burn those calories!), maintain normal blood pressure, and allow the brain to detoxify. So, what should you do? You can start by reducing caffeine and making an effort to turn the lights out by 10pm. Which means no smart phone, tablet, computer or television screen time at least an hour before bed. Next, create a nightly ritual and stick to it. Take a warm bath to relax, drink a cup of chamomile tea and tuck yourself in a few minutes early to journal or read a book. At first it may be difficult to fall asleep, especially if you've been a regular night owl. But if you stick with your new routine, it will become easier in time. Do the exercises in this book to reduce your stress and aim for 7 to 8 hours of sleep. Some woman swear by taking Melatonin or 5-HTP supplements. I like diffusing essential oils like Lavender or doTERRA's Serenity blend. Works wonders. Sweet dreams!

Eat Clean

What you put into your body is even more important than what you put on it. If you want to live a long and healthy life, you need to treat your body well. It's the only one you have after all! And food is life. Refer to my chapter on Clean Eats for healthy and nourishing recipes. My number one rule is to eat lots of plant based food. Make leafy greens a staple in your everyday menu and choose vegetables and fruits from the colors of the rainbow. By eliminating processed food and sugar, you will notice a surge in energy and clearer skin. Limit your grains to gluten free varieties like quinoa and brown rice. Eat clean protein at every meal and avoid dairy, alcohol, and soy. Have some healthy fats every day for your brain health.

Hydrate

We need water to survive! And many of us busy women don't drink nearly enough. Being dehydrated makes you feel tired and can even cause cravings. Your goal is to consume ½ your body weight in ounces of water every day. In other words, if you weighed 120 lbs., your goal would be to drink 60 ounces of water per day. Try to drink your water between meals and not while you are eating. An hour before or after works best for proper digestion.

Drink Lemon Water

I cannot live without my morning lemon water. Drinking warm water with fresh lemon juice, a teaspoon of raw apple cider vinegar, and a teaspoon of raw honey has been my ritual for the last two years. Lemons are cleansing, support the liver for proper detoxification and alkalize the body. I've noticed a huge difference in the way I feel once I started drinking my lemon elixir every morning. Oh, did I mention that lemons are great for making your skin glow!

Take Smart Supplements

Your very first source of nutrients should be from whole foods. However, as the body ages it becomes less efficient in making, absorbing, and storing certain vitamins and minerals. Plus, the soil today is not as rich in nutrients as it once was. These are the supplements that I take every day and recommend to all my clients over the age of 40.

- Omega 3 Fish Oil (purified to remove contaminants)
- Vitamin D3, 2,000 IU
- Coenzyme Q10, 100 mg
- Magnesium (citrate or chelate, <u>not</u> oxide) 350 mg
- Vitamin B-complex
- Protein Powder (Hemp or Pea, are my favorites)

Many women take a calcium supplement for bone health. Studies have shown that too much calcium isn't good, as the excess calcium is absorbed and stored in parts of your body where it can cause harm. If you want to take calcium supplements, I suggest not taking more than 300 mg twice a day. A very good source of calcium is by eating green leafy vegetables combined with a healthy fat.

Create a Mind-Body Practice

Having a mind-body practice is essential for healthy aging. I practice yoga, and it serves me perfectly. But if yoga is not your thing, any type of mindful movement will benefit you. You can try Qi Gong, Tai Chi, or a moving meditation exercise from this book. By having a mind-body practice, you are moving the energy (chi) throughout your body. In Chinese medicine, this is essential for maintaining perfect health. A mind-body practice is also wonderful for calming the mind and keeping your cortisol low.

Scrape Your Tongue

Yeah, I know, sounds weird. Based on Ayurveda practices, scraping the tongue helps keep bacteria and yucky plaque from building up in your mouth. I use a tongue scraper every morning after brushing my teeth. You can buy a tongue scraper at any health food store or online. Try it!

Create Meaningful Connections

As women, we are naturally more emotional than men. Which means we need the support of nurturing relationships in order to thrive. We enjoy the company of other women and we share our joy and sadness with our friends. I am very fortunate to have a group of women who have been in my life for over thirty five years. We get together often and have such great fun. Even if you don't live near your closest friends, you can meet some wonderful women and form strong friendships at any stage of your life. Potential friends are everywhere, through local mom's groups, school activities, neighbors, and your kid's extra-curricular activities. Just get out there and meet new people, stay connected and share some laughs!

Move Your Body

There seems to be a common trait that the older generation share. They move…a lot. Makes sense, right. Anyone over the age of 55 grew up without computers, iPads, Nintendo, Xbox, Facebook etc. Being a busy woman, I rarely sit down either. And now studies are showing a link between inactivity and a higher risk of heart disease. If you want to live a long life, keep moving. If you're at home watching television, get up during the commercials and walk around. Better yet, turn off the TV and head outside for a walk. If you don't like walking alone, get a dog. It works for me!

Spend Time in Nature

My favorite place to be. I love being among the trees, flowers, and mountains. I can feel my heart rate drop, my breath become deeper and my blood pressure go down. It's so incredibly healthy to be in the peacefulness of Mother Nature. If you don't live near a forest, a park, lake or anyplace undeveloped, it's time to take a road trip. Whatever place makes you feel peaceful will work. Just take time to get away from the concrete jungle. We need nature to *thrive*.

Drink Green Tea

Green tea is a potent antioxidant and will keep you looking young and staying healthy. Green tea contains polyphenols, a type of flavonoid which is proven to be potent enough to reduce the speed of cell aging. In fact, a flavonoid compound in green tea called EGCg has 20 times the potency of Vitamin C and Vitamin E, especially when it comes to reducing cell damage and aging. Just two cups a day is all you need!

Use Natural Personal Care Products

Guess what, everything we put on our bodies will absorb into our blood stream. To avoid chemicals and toxins, try to use natural soaps, skincare and hair care products whenever possible. Stay away from products with parabens, phalates, sulfates, triclosan, and other harmful chemicals. To check if your product is safe, use the skin deep database at www.ewg.org and look it up.

Be Adventurous!

Okay, so maybe you're not the type to go trekking in the Himalayas or rafting down the Amazon, but any kind of adventure will keep you feeling young. Do whatever feels exciting and fun for you!

"I think women should start to embrace their age. What's the alternative to getting older? You die. I can't change the day I was born. But I can take care of my skin, my body, and try to live my life and be happy."
— Olivia Munn

Chapter 16
Beyond Exercise

You probably already know that exercise is important for maintaining a healthy body. Whether you are running 5Ks or just working up to a twenty-minute walk around your neighborhood, it's important to move your body. But did you know that exercise aids in the release of toxins and is important for keeping the blood and lymphatic system flowing. Consistent exercise also helps to relieve stress by increasing blood flow to the brain. It stimulates the nervous system and releases endorphins into the body.

I have had some type of exercise routine nearly all of my life. It's something that makes me feel good, and if I happen to fall off track, I can feel a huge difference in my mood and energy. I always encourage my clients to find a form of exercise they enjoy, because if it's not fun you won't keep it up. Try walking, hiking, cycling, dancing, fitness videos, yoga, rebounding, or sign up for a group class at your gym. Just keep searching for something that keeps you motivated. Sometimes that means you have to switch it up once in a while, and that is perfectly fine! On the days that you feel too lazy to exercise, just put on your tennis shoes and walk for ten minutes. You might find that after ten minutes you are ready for more. Also, having a friend to exercise with can make it more fun, and you'll have a fitness buddy to keep you accountable.

Being active is also a wonderful mood enhancer. Exercise releases endorphins into your body, which makes you feel good and more positive. Of course, any kind of physical activity burns calories and helps to shed pounds, which I am guessing will also make you a happier person!

Top reasons people don't exercise:

- ✓ Not enough time
- ✓ Lack the self-motivation
- ✓ Don't like to exercise
- ✓ Find it boring
- ✓ Injured or have mobility limitations
- ✓ No support from family or friends
- ✓ Not close to walking trails

How to exercise and not step foot into a gym!

Go hiking
Go for a trail run
Ride a bike
Take a walk around the neighborhood
Dance to music in your living room
Take the stairs, always!
Chase your dog at the park
Try a hula hoop
Take Salsa lessons
Jump rope
Go swimming
Go kayaking
Try stand up paddle boarding
Run or walk on the treadmill at home
Use a mini trampoline (aka rebounder)
Park your car in the farthest spot and walk

Chapter 17
Stock a Nourishing Pantry

If your kitchen is healthy, then you will be healthy! Stocking your pantry with nutritious food is key to your success. If you have the right foods at your fingertips when hunger strikes, then you are more likely to eat it. Over the years my kitchen has become healthier and healthier. It may have taken a little longer than I wanted, because I live with a husband and child who didn't appreciate healthy food. But as I learned more about eating clean and how to cook with whole foods, my kitchen pantry eventually evolved. I'm happy to say my healthy food has finally won over 95% of the fridge and pantry. If you live with a more cooperative family, you may be able to do it even sooner!

Here are staple foods to keep in your healthy kitchen.

Grains and Pasta

Quinoa, buckwheat, millet and amaranth
Whole rolled or steel cut oats
Brown rice (not quick cooking)
Black (Forbidden) rice
100% whole grain pasta, look for quinoa and brown rice pasta
100% gluten-free tortillas
100% sprouted grain breads (Ezekiel bread is the preferred brand)

Legumes (Dried or canned, look for BPA free)

Black beans
Kidney beans
White beans
Lentils
Garbanzo
Adzuki beans

Nuts & seeds

Raw almonds and walnuts
Raw sunflower seeds
Raw, sliced almonds (for salads)
Raw pumpkin seeds
Flax seeds
Chia seeds
Nut butters; almond, cashew, sunflower seed

Produce (preferably organic)

Avocados
Any green vegetables (broccoli, Brussels sprouts, asparagus, cucumbers, green beans, zucchini etc.)
Red bell peppers
Carrots
Leafy greens (organic mixed greens, kale, spinach, chard, romaine, arugula)
Onions
Sweet potatoes
Lemons
Apples, grapes, bananas or your favorite snacking fruit
Blueberries, blackberries, strawberries
Fresh herbs, like basil, cilantro and chives
Garlic

Frozen Foods

Organic frozen berries
Assorted vegetables
Veggie burgers
Wild caught salmon fillets, prawns, halibut steaks

Animal Protein

Try to look for a local farm as they often have meats that are grass-fed and may not be certified organic but are treated humanely.

Organic or pastured eggs
Organic chicken and turkey breast
Nitrate-free bacon, turkey bacon
Nitrate-free deli meats
Organic grass-fed beef or bison
Wild caught Salmon, mackerel, sardines
Halibut, or other whole white fish

Beverages

Unsweetened almond milk
Unsweetened coconut milk
Coconut water
Green tea
Herbal teas such as chamomile, roasted dandelion root, rooibos, or peppermint

Oils (preferably cold-pressed)

Extra virgin olive oil
Sesame oil
Coconut oil
Avocado oil

Condiments and Vinegars

Aged balsamic vinegar
Red wine vinegar
Raw apple cider vinegar
Hummus
Tahini
Dijon mustard
Wheat-free tamari
Miso paste
Organic ketchup
Kim Chee
Raw Sauerkraut

Spice Cabinet

Cinnamon
Vanilla bean
Cayenne Pepper
Turmeric
Ginger powder
Basil
Oregano
Cumin
Sea Salt
Black Pepper

Chapter 18
Clean Eats Recipes

What does it mean to eat clean? Eating clean means making meals using fresh whole food. Unlike the Standard American Diet (SAD) which relies heavily on processed foods, unhealthy fat and too much sugar, you are eating a more plant based diet free of artificial anything. If a food has ingredients you can't pronounce, chances are it will create an imbalance in your gut flora. When I started to eat clean, my energy increased, my brain fog cleared up, and I felt incredible every day. Just the simple move to eliminate processed foods made a huge difference in my overall health.

Here's an interesting fact, about 95% of the hormone serotonin is made in the gut, making it even more important to keep our digestive system balanced. Serotonin is our happy, calm and content hormone, it keeps us feeling like the world is wonderful. Hormones are powerful and affect our mood, but they also affect our food choices. Ever wonder why you crave cookies and brownies when you feel sad? It's because carbohydrate-rich food promote production of serotonin.

But rather than reach for empty calories like processed snacks to make you feel good, why not keep your digestion healthy and balanced by eating clean foods. If your diet has consisted of mostly ready-made food, it may be challenging to find yourself spending more time in the kitchen. Don't be afraid, if you use my simple preparation tips, you will become a whiz at creating delicious and healthy meals in no time. Here are some of my favorite recipes, borrowed from my seasonal cleanses and my own personal recipe file. Enjoy!

Recipes

Smoothies

A perfect way to start your day, and great for lasting energy. Just throw all the ingredients into a high powered blender and blend! You can also add a scoop of hemp or pea protein powder for an extra boost of energy!

A Perfect Date

1 ½ cups unsweetened almond or coconut milk
2 Medjool dates, soaked and pitted
1 frozen banana
1 teaspoon cinnamon
1 teaspoon vanilla
1 tablespoon raw honey

Spiced Pumpkin Pie

1 cup unsweetened coconut or almond milk
½ cup pumpkin puree
½ teaspoon vanilla
½ frozen banana
¼ teaspoon pumpkin pie spice
¼ teaspoon cinnamon
1 tablespoon raw honey

Love My Smoothie

1 cup unsweetened coconut or almond milk
1 banana
1 tablespoon chia seeds
1 cup spinach
1 cup frozen berries
¼ teaspoon cinnamon
1 splash pure vanilla extract
Ice (optional)

Chocolate Heaven

1 cup almond or coconut milk
1 banana
2 tablespoons cashew butter
1 tablespoon raw honey
2 tablespoons unsweetened cocoa powder or raw cacao
Ice (optional)

Choco-berry

1 cup unsweetened almond or coconut milk
2 dates, soaked and chopped
1 tablespoon chia seeds
1 cup frozen berries of your choice
2 teaspoons raw cacao powder

Breakfasts

It's so important to start your day with a healthy breakfast! Whether you are having a smoothie or warm breakfast, you need to make sure your meal includes protein, healthy fat and fiber.

Warm Berry Chia Pudding

1 cup non-dairy milk
⅓ cup chia seeds
1 teaspoon raw honey
½ cup organic berries (raspberries, blueberries, strawberries)
½ teaspoon vanilla
Dash of cinnamon
Dash of ground ginger

In a small saucepan, add your non-dairy milk and vanilla and warm over a medium low flame. Make it hot, but not boiling.

While the milk is heating up, add your chia seeds to a cereal bowl. Sprinkle with the cinnamon and ground ginger. When the milk is ready, pour it over the chia seeds and mix thoroughly. Let sit for a few minutes to allow it to gel. Top your warm chia pudding with berries. Serve immediately.

Kim's Yummy Oatmeal

½ cup gluten free rolled oats
1 cup water
¼ cup coconut or almond milk
2 tablespoons toasted walnuts
2 tablespoons shredded coconut
¼ cup fresh blueberries
Cinnamon

Boil the water and add the rolled oats. Cook over low heat until water is absorbed. Add the milk and simmer for a few minutes. Transfer to a bowl and top with walnuts, coconut and blueberries. Sprinkle with cinnamon.

Breakfast Quinoa with Berries

1 cup quinoa
2 cups water
1 tablespoon coconut oil
1 tablespoon raw honey
¼ cup berries (blueberries, raspberries, strawberries)
Drizzle of coconut milk

Rinse the quinoa before cooking. Add the water and quinoa to a pot and cook according to package directions. While still warm, add coconut oil. Then add the raw honey. Add berries of your choice and drizzle coconut milk over the berries.

Eggs and Greens

2 organic eggs
1 cup chopped kale
½ cup chopped red bell pepper
½ cup sliced mushrooms
½ cup diced onions
1 tomato sliced
1 tablespoon coconut oil
¼ teaspoon turmeric
Sea salt and pepper to taste

Heat the oil in a skillet. Add the onions, peppers, and mushrooms and sauté a couple of minutes. Add kale and cook until wilted, about 5 to 10 minutes. Add chopped tomatoes and cook a couple minutes more. Season with salt, pepper, turmeric and dulse.

While the greens are cooking, poach your eggs in a separate pot. Serve the poached eggs on top of the cooked greens.

Super Seed Cereal

1 cup unsweetened vanilla almond milk
¼ cup sunflower seeds
¼ cup pumpkin seeds
¼ cup dried cranberries
2 tablespoons unsweetened shredded coconut
1 teaspoon cinnamon
1 teaspoon ground ginger
1 teaspoon raw honey

Slowly heat your milk in a saucepan for 2 or 3 minutes. Make it as hot as you can without boiling. Add the honey and stir.

In a bowl, add the sunflower seeds, pumpkin seeds, cranberries, cinnamon, ginger and coconut. Pour the warm milk over your mixture and enjoy!

Lunches

Veggie Ginger Nori Wraps

4 nori sheets
½ cup baby spinach leaves
¼ cup purple cabbage, chopped
¼ cup carrots, shredded
½ cup sprouts
1 small cucumber, sliced lengthwise
⅛ to ¼ bunch cilantro, chopped
2 to 3 one-inch pieces of ginger, cut in thin strips
½ avocado, sliced thin

Lemon Dijon Dressing
1 tablespoon Dijon mustard
1 tablespoon raw honey
1 tablespoon extra virgin olive oil
1 lemon, juiced
Sea salt to taste
Black pepper to taste

Add Dijon mustard, liquid sweetener, extra virgin olive oil, lemon juice, sea salt, and black pepper to a small bowl. Whisk until well incorporated. Set aside.

Lay out a nori sheet on a clean, dry surface. Layer your vegetables about 1 inch away from one of the sides. Take the 1-inch side and roll the nori sheet towards the opposite end. Try to roll it as tight as possible without tearing the sheet. When you roll the nori sheet to the end, place a drop of water on the end tips to keep it closed. Slice the wraps into one-inch pieces. Serve with lemon-mustard dressing.

(Adapted from Rachel Feldman www.rachelswellness.com)

Kale, Apple and Pumpkin Seed Salad

2 bunches of kale, small chiffonade
1/2 lemon, juiced
1 Fuji apple, cubed
1 tablespoon Dijon mustard
1/2 cup organic olive oil
2 Tablespoon honey
Splash of raw apple cider vinegar
1 cup pumpkin seeds
1/2 cup cranberries

Massage kale with lemon juice using your hands for three minutes to break it down.

In a smaller bowl, combine mustard, honey, vinegar and sea salt. While whisking mixture vigorously, add the organic olive oil slowly in a thin stream. Mix dressing with kale and top with pumpkin seeds, cranberries and apple.

Mediterranean Tuna

2 cans chunk light (or Skipjack) tuna
¼ cup chopped fresh cilantro
¼ cup chopped scallions
2 tablespoons extra virgin olive oil
1 tablespoon capers
1-2 tablespoons Dijon mustard (to taste)
1 tablespoon lemon juice
½ teaspoon finely grated lemon zest
Sea salt & pepper to taste

In a large mixing bowl, combine all of the ingredients. You can stuff it in bell peppers, wrap it up in lettuce, or add it on top of a mixed green salad.

(Adapted from Rachel Feldman www.rachelswellness.com)

Curried Quinoa Salad

3 cups cooked quinoa
¼ cup chopped onions
½ cup chopped red bell pepper
¼ cup raisins
¼ cup sliced almonds
¼ cup cilantro (chopped)
1 teaspoon curry powder
½ teaspoon turmeric

Cook quinoa according to the package directions. Transfer to a bowl and let cool in the refrigerator. When it's no longer warm, add the onions, bell peppers, raisins, curry powder and turmeric. Stir well and then add the cilantro and almonds.

Roasted Onion Soup

2 large onions, sliced
4 cloves garlic
4 cups of vegetable broth (organic)
1 tablespoon extra virgin olive oil
½ tablespoon dried thyme
Sea salt and pepper to taste
Splash of red cooking wine (optional)

Place your sliced onions and garlic in a large bowl. Massage with extra virgin olive oil. Place in a roasting pan and cook for 20 to 25 minutes at 400 degrees. Add the roasted onions and garlic to a large soup pot. Add the broth, thyme, sea salt and black pepper to the pot over medium high heat. Bring the soup to a boil and add the red cooking wine. Simmer for five minutes and serve.

Tasty Lentil & Kale Soup

2 cups vegetable broth
1 cup water
2 cups cooked lentils
1 cup chopped kale
½ cup sliced mushrooms
½ cup chopped leek
1 tablespoon yellow miso paste
1 tablespoon coconut oil

In a large pot, sauté the leeks and mushrooms in the coconut oil until soft. Add the broth, water and miso paste to the pot. Taste and add more miso if needed. Bring the broth to a light boil and then add kale and cooked lentils. Simmer for 15 minutes and serve.

Dinners

Sautéed Curry Veggies

1 pound cauliflower, broccoli, zucchini
1 yellow onion, diced
2 tbsp. coconut oil
6 oz. can tomato paste (look for a BPA FREE can)
½ can coconut milk
1 glove garlic
½ tsp. cumin
½ tsp. ginger
1 tsp curry
½ tsp. chili powder
1 tsp. sea salt

Wash and chop vegetables. Sauté onions and garlic in coconut oil. Add seasonings, tomato paste and coconut milk and stir until smooth. Add vegetables and simmer for 15 minutes.

Southwest Lime Salmon

1 pound wild caught salmon – 4 fillets
1 -2 tablespoons olive oil
2 limes, sliced in half
1 teaspoon sea salt
1 teaspoon chipotle powder

Preheat oven to 350°. Rinse salmon, pat dry and place on a metal baking sheet. Rub each fillet with olive oil. Squeeze the juice from one-half lime onto each fillet. Sprinkle fillets with salt and chipotle, then place a slice of lime on top of each fillet. Place salmon in the oven and cook for 8-12 minutes, depending on how well done you like your fish.

Thai Butternut Squash Soup

2 medium to large butternut squash
1 onion
1 carrot
2 cloves garlic
2 tbsp. coconut oil
5 cups vegetable broth
1 ½ cup coconut milk
½ -1 teaspoon red curry paste
1/3 cup cilantro
3 lime leaves
2 stalks lemon grass

Wash squash; bake halved squash at 350 for 45-50 minutes. In a large pot, sauté onions, carrot, and garlic in coconut oil. Add vegetable broth and coconut milk. Mix in red curry paste. Then add cooked and cubed squash, cilantro and blend well. Simmer with lime leaves and lemon grass for 20 minutes or more.

(Adapted from Rachel Feldman www.rachelswellness.com)

Chicken Bone Broth

A great soup for detoxification, building bone health and making your skin glow.

1 whole chicken (free range, organic if possible)
12 cups cold filtered water
2 tablespoons apple cider vinegar
1 large onion, roughly chopped
2 carrots, peeled and roughly chopped
4 stalks celery roughly chopped
2 zucchini
5 cloves garlic, roughly chopped
1 bunch parsley or cilantro

Cut the chicken into several pieces. It is best to have chicken that has bones and skin. Place chicken pieces into a large stainless steel stockpot, cover with the cold water, add vinegar and vegetables (except parsley), and let stand for 30 minutes.

Bring to a boil, remove scum that rises to the top, reduce heat and simmer for 6 to 24 hours. (If you are short on time, at least simmer for 3 hours.) The longer you cook the stock, the richer and more flavorful it will be. About 10 minutes before you're ready to turn it off, add the parsley. (This adds more minerals to the broth.) **You can also use a crockpot if you have one.**

Remove chicken pieces with a slotted spoon and refrigerate. (When they're cool, take the meat off the bones and store in zip-lock bags in the freezer for other recipes, such as soups, salads, enchiladas, sandwiches and curries.) Strain the broth into a large bowl and place in the refrigerator until the fat rises to the top and can be skimmed off.

Kim's Healing Soup

When I am sick with a cold or flu (which rarely happens) this is the soup that I like to make. Chock full of nutrients, this soup is great even when you're not sick.

4 cups organic chicken broth
1 cup chopped kale
1 cup asparagus, sliced into 1 inch pieces
1 parsnip, chopped
½ cup broccoli
½ cup cauliflower
1 inch piece of ginger
3 cloves crushed garlic

Add all the ingredients into a big stock pot. Cook at medium heat until all the vegetables are tender, about 20 minutes. Transfer to a blender or use an immersion blender to purée.

Desserts

Raspberry Mousse

²/₃ cup coconut milk
1 ¹/₃ cups frozen raspberries, thawed
2 tablespoons raw honey
¼ teaspoon pure vanilla
¼ cup virgin coconut oil

Add all of the ingredients to a food processor or high speed blender except the coconut oil and process until completely smooth. Then, add the coconut oil and process for 30 seconds more.

Chocolate Ice Cream

2 frozen bananas
Splash of coconut or almond milk
1 Tablespoon raw cacao powder

Let frozen bananas thaw a few minutes and then add all of the ingredients to a food processor or high powered blender and process until completely smooth. Add more milk if you desire a creamier texture.

Snacks and Dressings

Energy Balls

¾ cup pumpkin seeds
¾ cup sunflower seeds
4 chopped dates (soaked)
3 tablespoon flax meal
3 tablespoons coconut oil
½ cup unsweetened, shredded coconut
¼ cup raisins
1 tablespoon raw honey (optional)

Combine all ingredients (except for shredded coconut & raisins) in a food processor. Stir in raisins and then form mixture into balls about the size of a golf ball. Roll each ball in the shredded coconut to coat and then refrigerate until chilled.

Kale Chips

1 bunch kale, stems removed and leaves torn into 2-inch pieces
2 tablespoons avocado oil
1 tablespoon fresh lemon juice
Sea salt

Preheat oven to 250 degrees. In a large bowl, drizzle kale with oil, and lemon juice. Season with salt. Massage oil into leaves until evenly coated. Transfer to a rimmed baking sheet and bake for 20 minutes or until they look dry and crisp. Let cool completely. Store in an airtight container for up to 3 days.

Tahini Dressing

½ cup tahini
½ cup cilantro
1 clove garlic, minced
Juice of 1 lemon
¼ - ½ cup water
Sea Salt to taste

Stir together the tahini and lemon juice in a small bowl. Add the water until desired consistency is reached. Add the garlic and cilantro and blend well.

Simple Lemon Dressing

2 lemons, juiced
1 tablespoon fresh basil, finely chopped
½ cup cold pressed extra virgin olive oil
Sea salt and black pepper to taste

Combine all the ingredients together and serve over your salad greens.

About the Author

Kim Robinson Neto had a major life shift after surviving the stress of being a new mother while caring for her sick and elderly parents. After years of feeling depleted, anxious and tired, she made a choice to regain her health and her life. At age 49, she returned to school to study holistic health and nutrition and learned how to find a healthy balance. After healing her body and mind, she now enjoys sharing her holistic approach to wellness and helps other busy women find their own perfect balance. Kim leads seasonal cleanse and detox groups, works one on one with clients, and offers clean eating programs and workshops. She is an Institute for Integrative Nutrition™ Certified Health Coach with board certification by the (AADP) American Association of Drugless Practitioners, a charter member of the International Association of Health Coaches and member of The New Self-Health Movement. When Kim isn't talking or writing about "health" she loves to practice yoga, hike with her dog, play at the beach, dabble in jewelry design, and spend quality time with her son and family.

For more information about Kim's wellness programs and upcoming events, or to receive a free healthy living guide, visit: **www.simplewellnesswithkim.com**

Come join a community of busy women and moms supporting each other toward a healthier and happier life. Share your story and post your own personal tips. Check out the *Stop Surviving, Start Thriving* community page at:
www.facebook.com/womenthrivingnow

Find even more natural living and beauty tips on Kim's Facebook page at: **www.facebook.com/simplewellnesswithkim**

References

Web:

http://www.webmd.com/food-recipes/news/20130710/could-artificial-sweeteners-cause-weight-gain

http://articles.mercola.com/sites/articles/archive/2009/10/13/artificial-sweeteners-more-dangerous-than-you-ever-imagined.aspx

http://www.themindfulword.org/2012/buddhas-brain-interview-rick-hanson/

http://greatergood.berkeley.edu/

http://sacramento.cbslocal.com/2013/03/04/study-female-brains-are-smaller-than-male-brains-but-used-more-efficiently/

http://www.responsibletechnology.org/gmo-dangers/65-health-risks/1notes

http://bodyecology.com/articles/one-weight-loss-mistake-you-dont-know-youre-making#.VOdoUfnF83k

http://kripalu.org/article/274

http://bodyecology.com/articles/interrupted-sleep-may-be-damaging-your-brain#.VO_LtvnF83k

http://www.scientificamerican.com/article/gut-second-brain/

Books:

Herbert Benson, MD, *The Relaxation Response* (New York: HarperTorch: Harper Collins Publishers, 1975)

AnneMarie Colbin, PhD, *Whole Food Guide to Strong Bones* (Oakland: New Harbinger Publications, 2009)

William Davis, MD, *Wheat Belly* (New York: Rodale, Inc., 2011)

Joel Fuhrman, MD, *Eat to Live* (New York: Little, Brown and Company, Revised 2011)

Sara Gottfried, MD, *The Hormone Cure* (New York: Scribner, 2013)

Rick Hanson, PH.D., Richard Mendius, MD, *Buddha's Brain: The Practical Neuroscience of Happiness, Love and Wisdom* (Oakland: New Harbinger Publications, 2009)

Jane Ogden, *Health Psychology: A textbook, 3rd edition.* (Open University Press - McGraw-Hill Education, 2004) p. 259.

David Perlmutter, MD, *Grain Brain: The Surprising Truth About Wheat, Carbs, and Sugar – Your Brain's Silent Killers* (New York: Little, Brown and Company, 2013)

JJ Virgin, CNS, CHFS, *JJ Virgin's Sugar Impact Diet* (New York: Grand Central Life & Style, 2014)

Dr. Libby Weaver, *Rushing Woman's Syndrome* (Little Green Frog Publishing Ltd., 2011)

Dr. Claudia Welch, MSOM, *Balance Your Hormones, Balance Your Life* (Philadelphia: Da Capo Press: Perseus Book Group, 2011)

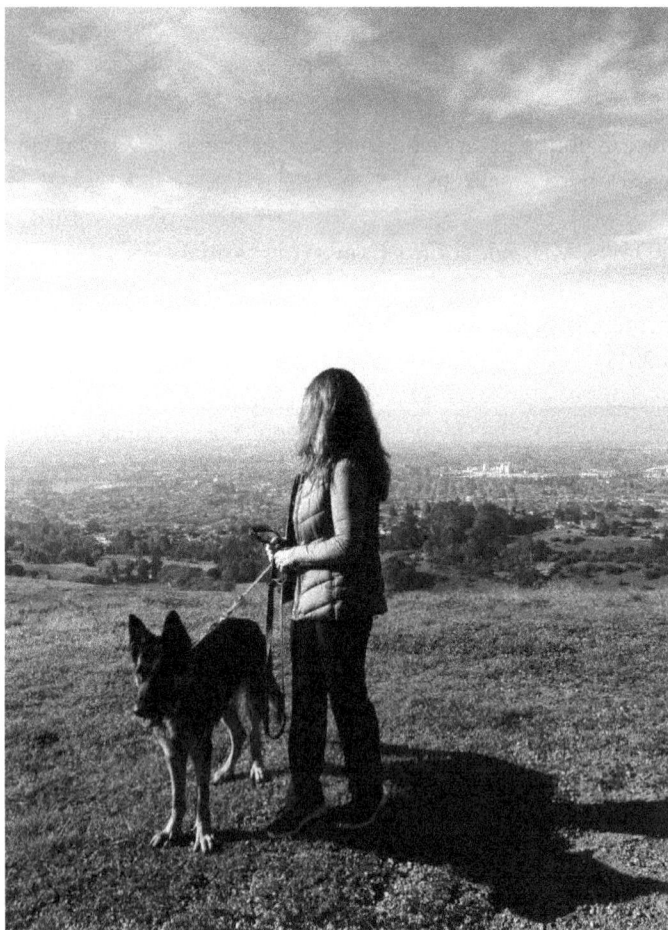

Photo credit: Alpana Aras-King

The author on a morning walk with her dog, Lobo.

My Notes

My Notes

My Notes

My Notes